Treating Acne and Rosacea
with Chinese Herbal Medicine

Treating Acne and Rosacea with Chinese Herbal Medicine

Sabine Schmitz

Foreword by Dan Bensky

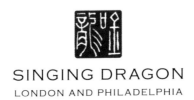

SINGING DRAGON

LONDON AND PHILADELPHIA

First published in Great Britain in 2022 by Singing Dragon,
an imprint of Jessica Kingsley Publishers
An Hachette Company

1

Copyright © Sabine Schmitz 2022
Foreword copyright © Dan Bensky 2022

Disclaimer: The information contained in this book is not intended to replace
the services of trained medical professionals or to be a substitute for medical
advice. The complementary therapy described in this book may not be suitable for
everyone to follow. You are advised to consult a doctor before embarking on any
complementary therapy programme and on any matters relating to your health, and
in particular on any matters that may require diagnosis or medical attention.

A CIP catalogue record for this title is available from the
British Library and the Library of Congress

ISBN 978 1 78775 227 6
eISBN 978 1 78775 228 3

Printed and bound in China by Leo Paper Products

Jessica Kingsley Publishers' policy is to use papers that are natural, renewable and recyclable
products and made from wood grown in sustainable forests. The logging and manufacturing
processes are expected to conform to the environmental regulations of the country of origin.

Jessica Kingsley Publishers
Carmelite House
50 Victoria Embankment
London EC4Y 0DZ

www.singingdragon.com

Dedicated to Steve Clavey! I appreciate your knowledge, your generosity and your constantly willingness to help. Beyond that, I love your sense of humour.

Serve others as best as you can! But never forget that in order to take good care of others, you should first take good care of yourself. Only a healthy and serene therapist is a good therapist. Stay away from greed, greed for wealth, compliments and fame. All of this is very irrelevant and does not contribute to health and happiness.

Sabine Schmitz

Contents

Foreword

SABINE SCHMITZ is a well-known practitioner who has trained both in East Asia and the West. Her *Treating Acne and Rosacea with Chinese Herbal Medicine* is an excellent example of how this type of practitioner can put together their varied experiences and learning into something that combines the best of the various approaches and mindsets that they have learned over the course of their studies and clinical practice. This gives a depth, an immediacy, and a liveliness to the text, and not only makes the information easier to read and to understand, but adds to its utility. In this work, the flexibility and responsiveness to the patient and the particular situation, which is the hallmark of efficacy when practicing traditional East Asian Medicine, comes through loud and clear.

This is the second of Sabine Schmitz's comprehensive and clinically useful books on subjects within the specialty of dermatology. This time the subject is acne and she utilizes all the facets of her integrated approach which includes both biomedical and traditional Chinese concepts. Integration in *Treating Acne and Rosacea with Chinese Herbal Medicine* is not just a catch phrase but baked into the book itself. It includes a dive into how the skin is seen both in Traditional Chinese Medicine and biomedicine, as well as an overview of how acne is viewed in biomedicine, the Chinese tradition, and modern TCM. The discussion of herbal treatment, although rooted in a Chinese medical perspective, also includes information on the pharmacological understanding of the most commonly used herbs, primarily as a tool to facilitate communication with patients and conventional practitioners, but it is also interesting for its own sake.

Some of the more practical aspects of this book include how to utilize various forms of Chinese medicinal treatments, such as decoctions, granules, tinctures, washes, wet compresses, and creams. This will help practitioners who did not learn this kind of thing in their studies to get the best results and also allow for more self-care on the part of patients. Similarly, there is a good section on the role of diet and lifestyle modifications in the treatment of acne.

The core of the book is the section on proper differentiation of various forms of acne and their appropriate treatment. This is done quite systematically, but not in a rigid manner. Additionally, Sabine has put in many different types of tips to help practitioners understand their patients' situation better as well as get better results. Some of these, such as paying attention to the emotional, environmental, and dietary circumstances of the patient, should be basic knowledge, but are often ignored. This is another example of how Sabine's dedication to the craft and experience in meeting patients where they are come through clearly in this text.

Dan Bensky
Seattle, January 2021

Acknowledgments

I WOULD LIKE TO thank my beloved dermatology teacher in China, my former tutor Professor Mǎ Lìlì. Without her knowledge and expertise, my work in Chinese dermatology would certainly not be the same. Yáng Zǐ and Fāng Yīmiào, faithful friends, deserve recognition for their generous and continuous support, be it in the translations from Chinese to English (and vice versa) or the collection of patient pictures. Thank you for always being there for me. I would also like to recognize my dear colleague Mary-Jo Bevin for conscientiously editing and proofreading my manuscript. I like it when you are strict and I love working with you! Finally, I offer my gratitude to Claire Wilson from Singing Dragon for believing in this new book series on TCM dermatology. I appreciate your support and that of the whole team at Singing Dragon, and am excited to continue working with you. But mostly I would like to thank my husband, Hans, for his continuous support and understanding in times when I did not have much time. I thank you for the last 23 years and I am sure you can do another 23 years with me and even more!

Disclaimer

THE INFORMATION in this book is given to the best of the author's knowledge. However, the author cannot be held responsible for any error or omission. The author disclaims any responsibility for any injury and/or damage to persons or property in connection with the use of the material contained in this book. Chinese medicine is professional medicine and this is a specialist book. The author does not advocate or endorse self-medication by laypersons. Laypersons interested in availing themselves of the treatment described in this book are advised to seek out a qualified professional practitioner of Chinese medicine. It is the responsibility of the treating physician to determine the method, the dosages of each therapeutic drug, and duration of treatment for the patient.

About the Author

SABINE SCHMITZ (M. Med. TCM) is a graduate of the Zhèjiāng Chinese Medical University in Hángzhōu, China, where she majored in Chinese medical dermatology. Her vast treasures of knowledge from China and her many years of clinical experience benefit numerous patients with chronic and complex skin diseases, as well as many patients with other diseases. Earlier in her career, Sabine worked in hospitals, laboratories, universities, and national and international clinical research for 15 years. Sabine is based in Cologne, Germany, and has a busy Traditional Chinese Medicine (TCM) practice specializing in skin diseases, gynecological disorders, and infertility treatment. She mainly works with Chinese herbal medicine and acupuncture.

Sabine is the founder and owner of CHINAMED COSMETICS (www.chinamed-cosmetics.com), an exciting range of modern natural herbal cosmetics based on the principles of TCM and made in Germany to high standards. She has developed a unique herbal formula providing an effective natural solution for anti-aging facial skincare.

Preface

THIS PRACTICAL HANDBOOK is the second in a series on dermatological diseases and their treatment with Chinese herbal medicine and deals with one of the most common skin conditions: acne vulgaris (acne). This book aims to be a comprehensive and helpful guide on Traditional Chinese Medicine (TCM) and acne in your daily practice.

The fact that skin diseases are a very broad field of expertise in TCM does not make it easier to treat them if you are not a specialist. This book zooms in on one of the most common skin conditions of today: acne. Its main purpose is to advise TCM professionals how to treat patients with acne in their daily practice. This comprehensive guide includes:

- basic information on the skin and its functions

- theoretical knowledge on the Western perception of acne

- detailed background information on the TCM perspective on acne throughout the past centuries

- thorough explanations of the most common TCM syndromes

- prescriptions and treatment options for all types of acne and TCM syndromes

- numerous case studies

- high-quality color images of the skin and tongue for precise diagnosis

- a full chapter on acne rosacea

- helpful advice on diet, lifestyle, skincare, and patient communication

- pharmacological properties of the most commonly used Chinese herbs in the treatment of acne

- a comprehensive section on how to make external applications such as pastes, washes, or ointments.

This text is designed as a practical and easy-to-understand manual that can be used immediately in everyday practice. It is neither a dry standard text nor a restating of existing literature. In this book, I pass on the knowledge I have gained in China and through my practical experience. I also provide many extra practical hints, because I strongly believe that these extras that are not usually included in the standard therapy are an essential part of clinical success.

Specialization in medical fields has become routine for good reason, and this also applies to Chinese medicine. Expert knowledge is crucial in understanding diseases at their core, and in treating them more specifically and thus more successfully. It is therefore not surprising that there is a high degree of specialization in the home country of TCM. I had the chance to learn the basics of TCM dermatology from my renowned teacher, Professor Mǎ Lìlì, in Hángzhōu, China. My studies under her and my work with her provided a profound basis, to which I have been able to add many years of experience with practical cases in my specialized practice. One important observation is that skin diseases are often complicated and neither easy nor fast to treat. I feel it is important to share this knowledge because I understand how difficult it is to learn TCM dermatology. Added to this are two factors: training is very rare and specialization is not as popular in the West. This is one of the main reasons that I am writing this book: to share much needed knowledge and expertise with my colleagues.

Is this book *Treating Acne and Rosacea with Chinese Herbal Medicine* for you? It is aimed at TCM professionals or students of TCM with a basic understanding of TCM. It will be useful for everyone who sees and treats skin diseases in their daily practice regardless of their specialization. I invite you to seize this opportunity and expand your knowledge on TCM, the skin, and acne in all its forms. You will be able to apply the knowledge you will gather from this book immediately and start treating your patients suffering from various forms and degrees of severity of acne with Chinese herbal medicine, in a way that is completely natural, long-lasting, and almost without side effects when properly applied.

The need for natural but effective and sustainable treatment methods definitely exists—you and I know this from our daily practice. Here, this demand meets a medicine that can draw on thousands of years of experience. This is why it is high time that TCM handbooks became available in English, reflecting the publications in numerous medical disciplines of Western medicine. To meet this need, this is the second handbook of a new TCM dermatology series exploring the most common skin diseases that I am working on with Singing Dragon. I want to create the ultimate resources for practitioners to use in clinical practice—easy to read, use, and navigate in day-to-day practice, and based on my experience of over a decade in treating skin conditions with Chinese medicine.

Introduction

S KIN CONDITIONS are a highly interesting and very complex topic. In the Western world, they are often perceived as a beauty issue and the market targeting people with skin problems is a multi-billion-dollar industry. However, many patients suffer from severe and usually chronic skin diseases. The major issue here is not only that these conditions are often difficult to treat but they also seriously affect patients' quality of life in multiple dimensions. This includes discomfort due to their appearance, scarring,[1] and emotional or psychosocial stress. As one of the most common skin diseases, acne is a perfect example of the way in which skin diseases seem to be an endless, inescapable fate. Acne affects approximately 9.4%[2] of the global population,[3] is often regarded as a "beauty problem," and can be hard to identify and treat.

Of course, we all know acne. Nearly everyone is affected by an outbreak at some time or other, perhaps after consuming aggravating foods or due to travel to different climatic conditions, which sometimes can have a negative impact on the skin–hot and humid regions, for example, can have this effect. Certainly, acne in teenagers is common. At the age of 13, nobody is surprised by blackheads, blemished skin, or acne. Skin blemishes in puberty are both a nuisance and a normal fact of teenage life as hormone levels are fluctuating wildly. But at a certain point there should be an end to pimples and inflamed, greasy skin, right? Unfortunately, the reality looks different. Many patients over the age of 30 also suffer from skin blemishes and late-onset acne. We need to clearly distinguish between blemished skin, acne in puberty, and adult acne. In this book, I primarily talk about acne in adults, as this represents the majority of patients I see in practice. However, this book is also useful for practitioners who treat teenagers, as–according to TCM–the skin is always treated according to the corresponding TCM pattern, which is independent of age, gender, or other distinctions.

A clear complexion is a sign of beauty in our society. And, no matter their age, most people want to feel beautiful or at least be comfortable in their own skin. When a glance in the mirror is a constant reminder that their appearance, especially in cases of very bad acne, does not fulfill common beauty standards, it really impacts the patient's self-confidence and, yes, their vanity. Sure, there is an entire market sector targeting these people, but despite what advertising suggests, although cosmetic products might be able to cover some of the blemishes, anyone who has ever seen a very serious case of deep acne knows that there is no hiding it. Plus, there are scars that remain, as well as itching or pain. Therefore, dealing with acne on a daily basis is not easy and patients definitely need our help (as they do with all skin diseases).

Acne mainly occurs in very exposed areas of the body–usually on the face where it can be seen by everyone. It affects both men and women. Regardless of gender, people are often ashamed and usually spend a lot of money and time on expensive cosmetic products or procedures that do not help–and if they do help, it is only temporary. The problem is that patients often feel under pressure to improve their skin condition, and, according to TCM, this does not make the situation any better. On the contrary, any form of pressure causes stress, which makes the qi stagnate. The interplay of emotions and skin conditions is discussed in Chapter 4. This much can be said right away, however: Pressure or frustration always interferes with the free qì dynamic. Blocked qì that can no longer move freely and thus stagnates within the body always tends to produce heat after some time, if there is no intervention. This mechanism is not uncommon in patients with acne and they must be aware of this vicious cycle. We, as their TCM doctors, should explain the process and give them the chance to do the work on themselves. Letting go of expectations and pressure on themselves is essential for our treatment. We need to communicate that the patient is always part of the therapy. This is why this book provides a lot of useful practical information for both TCM practitioners and their patients.

Clinical experience shows that stress, environment, and nutrition play a very important role in the development of acne. This book addresses and discusses all these factors (see Chapter 4). In my practice, patients often tell me that they have read–mostly on the internet–that a healthy diet can cure skin diseases. As true as this might be with occasionally blemished skin, it is certainly not possible to cure complex skin diseases with dietary changes alone. Patients are often incredibly disappointed if they follow a strict diet and then do not achieve the promised effect. Although nutrition is a very important part of the treatment, it is not the sole solution. Emotions and life circumstances play an equally important role. And there is a complex physical system, in which the skin reflects our well-being. This is where TCM can help.

Usually, patients with acne first see a Western dermatologist and/or cosmetician–and, from my experience, in most cases not just one. There, they are prescribed either unhelpful creams that deal with blemishes on the surface or antibiotics as pills or topical cream. The latter, of course, does not make any sense when we consider that in many cases the cause is rooted inside the body. Plus, oral antibiotics may cause severe side effects.[4] Any administration of this kind of medication should be extremely conservative. As benefits should always outweigh the risks, it simply seems unreasonable to give antibiotics to acne patients. Another option Western dermatologists often take is to prescribe patients chemical exfoliating agents[5] over a very long period of time, which irritates the skin even more. In addition, many patients complain of feeling neglected and ill-informed. At the end of this ordeal, patients start looking for other treatment options to help their skin. TCM offers this help with a completely different approach: precise, individually targeted, and natural. The advantage of TCM is that each patient receives her or his individual treatment plan, including internal and/or external treatment, always adapted to their individual needs and flexibly modified at every visit. This approach has proven to be helpful for many patients with acne.

The book begins with a theoretical discussion and background information about acne, detailing the most common types of acne, its causes, and current treatment options in Western medicine, accompanied by many pictures and illustrations. The second part of the book is a hands-on practical guide looking at the root cause of acne from a Chinese medicine viewpoint, examining the most common Chinese medicine syndromes, and presenting formulas that have been proven to be most effective with both internal and external applications of herbal medicine (see Chapter 3). Many pictures of the skin and tongue accompany each TCM syndrome, for easy reference in your daily practice. The role of diet, environment, and emotional health is elaborated on in detail in Chapter 4. In addition to this, for better understanding and providing assistance in your practice, a separate chapter on acne rosacea is included.

This book takes a modern, practical approach to treatment, and I hope it will serve as a comprehensive resource for practitioners to use in clinical practice–accessible, useful, and easy to navigate in day-to-day practice. I sincerely hope that many more patients will experience how TCM can enhance their quality of life.

Endnotes

1 Scarring is quite a common phenomenon after severe and deep acne has abated.

2 Acne vulgaris. *Vulgaris* is the medical term for "common" (common acne). Non-medical persons may prefer to call acne "pimples" or "spots."

3 Tan, J.K.L. and Bhate, K. (2015) "A global perspective on the epidemiology of acne." *British Journal of Dermatology 172*, Suppl. 1, 3–12.

4 In TCM, antibiotics are considered to be very cool. It is said that they are believed to cool and weaken the Spleen qì and yáng in the first place, but also lead to the production of dampness in many cases. This can either be due to the weakening of Spleen qì and yáng or due the inhibition of the intestinal peristalsis. Source: Ritter, S. (2016) *Arzneimittelwirkungen aus Sicht der Chinesischen Medizin*. München: Verlag Müller & Steinicke.

5 Chemical peeling substances such as alpha hydroxy acid, salicylic acid, glycolic acid, or vitamin A acid, for instance–also called keratolytics.

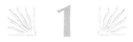

The Skin

B EFORE TREATING a skin disease, it is crucial to know the anatomical structure and functions of the skin. This way, we can understand better how dysfunction develops, the role individual components play, and finally how to treat skin diseases such as acne successfully.

The Anatomical Structure of the Skin

With a surface area of 1.5–2.0 m², the skin is the largest organ of our body. It is also the most vulnerable organ–and clearly visible in its vulnerability. This is certainly one of the reasons why patients are often quite frustrated or even depressed when they experience changes on their skin: They and (on some body parts) everyone else can clearly see unhealthy skin. Many patients feel uncomfortable and ashamed, in particular if acne is located in the face–which, of course, it is most of the time. Patients cover up pimples with make-up or powder, but although that might help appearance-wise to some extent, it does not treat the problem in itself. Usually, make-up simply clogs the pores even more–exactly one of the things to be avoided with acne.

The skin forms the interface between an individual and their environment. It is the body's primary barrier against microbial pathogens and, thus, protects us every day. The skin also contains adnexal structures such as hair, nails, and sweat glands, as well as vessels, nerves, melanocytes, and the skin-associated immune system.

The skin has three layers: the epidermis, the dermis, and the subcutaneous fatty region. Each layer performs specific tasks, which will be described below.

Epidermis

The epidermis, relatively thin and tough, acts as the shield for the body. It is an external elastic layer that continuously regenerates every 28–30 days. The epidermis is composed of highly specialized epithelial cells, known as keratinocytes, which are arranged into multiple layers. They are continuously replenished from just one layer of basal keratinocytes, which divide frequently. Dead skin cells called corneocytes form the uppermost layer, which is largely responsible for the skin's barrier function. Scattered throughout the basal layer of the epidermis are cells called melanocytes. They synthesize the pigment melanin, the main photo-protective factor, which also gives our skin its color.

Other epidermal cells are: Langerhans cells, the antigen-presenting immune cells of the skin; and Merkel cells, the neuroendocrine cells that function as mechanoreceptors essential for light touch sensation. They are mainly found in sensitive skin regions–for example, the fingertips and tip of the nose.

Dermis

The dermis is the layer beneath the epidermis, and it is the major structural component of the skin. In the dermis, the predominant cells are fibroblasts. They secrete elastin and collagen fibers that form a dense extracellular matrix. This extracellular matrix gives the skin its flexibility and strength. The dermis contains nerve endings, sweat glands and sebaceous glands, hair follicles, blood and lymph vessels, as well as mast cells. Blood vessels nourish the dermis, while lymphatic fluid is drained through the lymph vessels to the lymph nodes. Blood vessels also help regulate the temperature by dilating or contracting, which is why the skin pales when a person feels cold and reddens when he or she flushes.

Subcutis (Hypodermis)

Between the dermis and the muscle fascia lies the subcutaneous tissue, a layer of fat that helps insulate the body from heat and cold, provides protective padding for shock absorption, and allows the storage of fat for energy reserves. The fat remains in adipose (fat) cells, held together by fibrous tissue. It is surrounded by connective tissue, larger blood vessels, and nerves. The fatty layer varies in thickness, from very thin on the eyelids to several centimeters on the abdomen and gluteal region in some people.

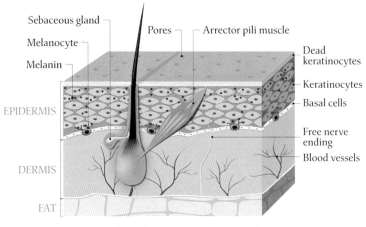

THE ANATOMY OF THE SKIN[1]

The Physiological Functions of the Skin

The skin performs a number of important functions. As the interface between the body and the environment, it plays a key role in protecting the body against external pathogens, and forms a barrier for the exchange of fluids. Other functions are temperature control, sensation, and communication.

Protection

Due to the keratinization of the epithelium and glandular secretions, the skin forms an anatomical barrier against pathogens and damage. The skin serves as the body's defense system to the external environment. It protects the body against mechanical, chemical, and thermal damage. It also protects the body against the invasion of external microorganisms.

Immune Response

The skin is a dynamic organ and also participates in the body's immune-biological defense processes. It contains different cells, such as the Langerhans cells, which are part of the adaptive (acquired) immune system and are activated when the tissue is under attack by invading pathogens. Memory T cells patrol the skin and are capable of responding to repeated attack from the outside, by monocytes and mast cells. Memory T cells are T cells that have learned how to fight off an invader by "remembering" the strategy used to defeat previous infections. This mechanism is particularly important in gaining life-long immunity to infections such as scarlet fever, rubella, mumps, or chickenpox.

Temperature Control

Temperature control is the process of keeping the body at a constant temperature of 37°C. Sweat regulation and skin blood flow are both essential for maintaining the body's core temperature. Sweating begins almost precisely at a skin temperature of 37°C and increases rapidly as the skin temperature rises above this value, regulated by neural feedback mechanisms which operate primarily through the hypothalamus.[2] If skin temperature drops below 37°C, a variety of responses are initiated to preserve heat within the body and to increase heat production. These include vasoconstriction to decrease the flow of heat to the skin and the cessation of sweating.

Water Resistance

The skin also acts as a barrier to water. Skin barrier function depends on the lipid-enriched stratum corneum cell membrane in the epidermis. Water resistance is important because it prevents the body from losing essential nutrients and minerals.

Sensation

Another important function of the skin is detecting the different sensations of heat, cold, touch, pressure, vibration, tissue injury, and pain. Sensation is felt through a rich network of nerve endings with a variety of sensory receptors in the dermis.

Synthesis of Vitamin D

Vitamin D is crucial for building and maintaining strong bones. The synthesis of vitamin D is induced by ultraviolet (UV) light and is then transmuted in the liver and in the kidneys into a hormone called calcitriol. Calcitriol increases the blood calcium level by promoting the absorption of dietary calcium from the gastrointestinal tract into the blood. Calcitriol also stimulates the release of calcium from the bones. It thus affects the human bone's mineral density and bone turnover. Vitamin D deficiency causes osteomalacia, called rickets when it occurs in children.

Absorption and Excretion

Although the skin is a waterproof barrier, some substances such as certain drugs and remedies can be administered through the skin by means of ointments or adhesive patches and essential oils. Those substances can penetrate the skin through the layers, the hair follicles, and sweat glands. The extent of penetration is limited by the skin's health and condition.

The skin serves as an excretory organ, disposing of waste material and toxins. Waste substances are expelled from the body through the skin via the sweat glands and normally take the form of salts, carbon dioxide, urea, and ammonia.

If all these tasks are performed properly, our skin is healthy and resilient. We are warmed and protected. The complexion looks bright and there are no pathological changes. We simply look good.

The Natural Skin Surface Potential of Hydrogen (pH)

It might be surprising that the natural potential of hydrogen (pH) on the surface of the skin is below 5 on average, which is beneficial for its resident flora. An acidic pH (4–4.5) keeps the skin healthy: it prevents the growth of bacteria and fungi, and thus protects the outer layers of the skin. In contrast, with an alkaline pH (8–9) important skin fats for the protective acid mantle can no longer build up. The skin loses water, dries out, and is no longer able to offer sufficient protection. Alkaline substances can no longer be neutralized and the skin becomes vulnerable to infection. In acne, a pH shift is rather typical. Thus, bacteria (*P. acnes*)[3] grow and result in an inflammation of the skin. Note, that not all germs are bad as such. Commensal microbes, such as bacteria, viruses, and fungi living on the skin, have beneficial effects in the protection against pathogens and facilitate wound healing. In a healthy balance, they form a perfect symbiosis to protect us. It is their imbalance–as is commonly the case with imbalances–that is harmful.

Here is a good example of *P. acnes* having infected the skin. In this patient's case, the skin was examined with a Wood's lamp which uses transillumination (light) to detect bacterial or fungal skin infections. This test is also known as the black light test or the ultraviolet light (UV) test. The light is held over an area of skin in a darkened room. Changes in the skin's pigmentation or the presence of certain bacteria or fungi will cause the affected area to change color under the light. This means the UV light will cause the organisms to fluoresce, as can be seen in the pictures.

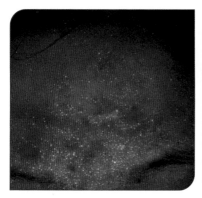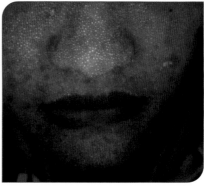

The skin, as our largest organ, carries great responsibility for our well-being. It protects us every single day. It literally holds us together. This is why it is essential to treat it well. A big problem is excessive personal hygiene, such as showering too often or with water that is too hot, using masses of shower gel, or, even worse, shower gel which contains chemicals, irritating substances, and perfumes. Visits to a solarium or using chemicals to make the skin looked tanned, which might have a positive visual effect at first, are not a good way to take care of our skin in the long run. These habits harm our skin, which then is no longer able to sustain its natural function as a barrier: the skin becomes irritated, inflamed, or so dried out that it can no longer be nourished. Therefore, patients often need to reconsider their skin routines. It can be helpful to advise patients to use mild and pH-neutral shower gels without perfume–the best choice for sensitive skin anyway. Most of all, however, we need to create awareness that not only is the skin highly sensitive to internal and external factors, but its functions as an organ are crucial for our well-being.

Endnotes

1   Source: Adapted from Shutterstock.

2   The hypothalamus is an important "control center" of our body. It is an area of the brain in the interbrain (diencephalon) and it is located below (= hypo) the thalamus. The hypothalamus contains not only control mechanisms for water, salt balance, and blood pressure, for instance, but also the key temperature sensors. It is also an important inceptor within the endocrine system because it regulates the timing and quantity of hormonal formation.

3   *Propionibacterium acnes.*

2

The Western View of Acne

The Etiology of Acne According to Western Medicine

In Western medicine, the pathogenesis of acne is multifactorial. And these factors vary with age. Often, the sebaceous glands are increasingly active, not uncommonly hormone-induced, due to disturbed follicular keratinization and microbial interactions. This might be due to a genetic predisposition,[1] hormonal changes, or lifestyle factors such as unhealthy nutrition or smoking,[2] but it could also be elicited by stress or even the wrong cosmetic products, insufficient hygiene, or sun damage. A frequent issue is that people secretly (and excessively) pick or squeeze outbreaks, or conceal them with make-up instead of addressing the main causes of impure skin and pimples: excessive sebum production and hyperkeratinization (the accumulation of dead skin cells).

This is how the problem develops. The primary lesion is usually a comedone (blackhead), a clogged hair follicle (pore) in the skin. If excess sebum cannot drain, bacteria can easily colonize and cause inflammatory foci. Thus, nodules of different sizes and depths and pus-filled pustules easily arise. Countermeasures such as frequent washing or strong chemical degreasing products for cleaning actually destroy the natural skin barrier and thus promote cornification and even further sebum congestion. Although Western medicine tries to interrupt this vicious cycle, the approaches and results seen in practice are often anything but satisfactory. Moreover, as Western medicine is usually a symptom-related treatment, there are many relapses with skin issues such as acne. In contrast, TCM approaches treatment differently and always assesses the skin condition that an individual patient presents with as part of an underlying condition.

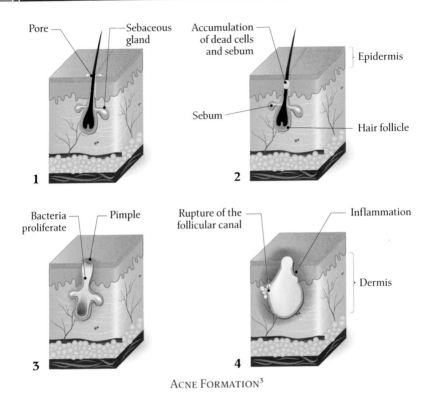

ACNE FORMATION[3]

The Most Common Types of Acne

Acne vulgaris, commonly referred to as acne, can occur on various parts of the body, including the face, neck, chest, shoulders, and arms. However, there are many overlapping types of acne. Here are the most common types of acne breakouts.

Whiteheads

This is a mild form of acne that appears as small, round, white bumps on the skin's surface. Whiteheads occur when sebum and dead skin cells prevent a clogged hair follicle from opening. If this clogged hair follicle is covered with a thin layer of skin, the surface appears white.

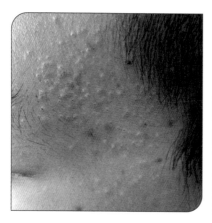

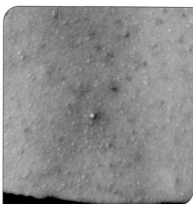

Acne Papulosa

Papules are comedones[4] that become inflamed and appear as small red or pink raised bumps on the skin. This type of pimple can be sensitive and painful.

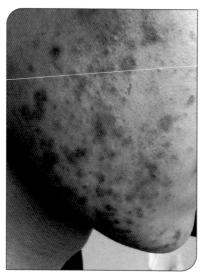

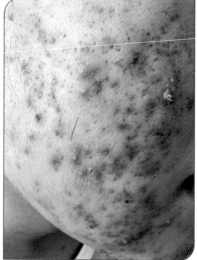

Acne Pustulosa

Pustules are inflamed pimples that are typically filled with white or yellow pus. Squeezing can lead to scars or dark spots on the skin.

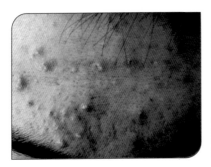
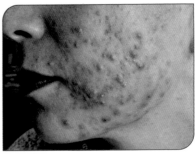

Acne Nodosa

This is a severe form of acne that develops deep under the skin. The nodules are large, and generally do not contain pus, but are hard and often very painful.

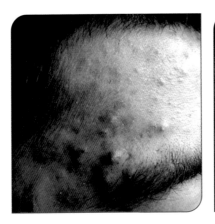
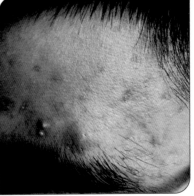

Acne Nodulocystica

Nodulocystic acne, a severe form of acne, has multiple inflamed cysts and nodules due to bacteria invading the blocked pore. The lesions may turn deep red or purple and often leave scars. This form of acne is very difficult to treat, both in Western medicine and in TCM.

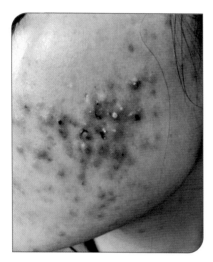 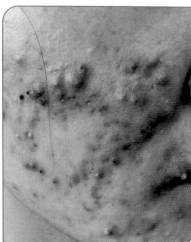

Acne Cystica

The pure form of cystic acne, another severe form of acne in which cysts are large and the pus-filled lesions look similar to boils, is very rare and not commonly seen in a TCM practice.

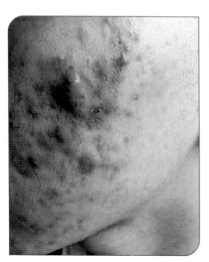 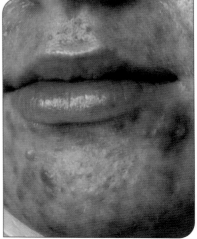

Two Special Types of Acne
Acne Inversa

This type of acne is not very common, but practitioners should know its features and make a precise diagnosis as it can be often improved or even cured with TCM.

Acne inversa, also known as hidradenitis suppurativa (HS), occurs chronically and in spurts. Deep pimples and inflammation can occur in one or multiple areas of the body and usually develop in the armpits, groin, and anal area. This type causes long-term skin inflammation and can be very painful. Patients often report surgical excision, often in combination with antibiotics, corticosteroids, or topical vitamin A-based drugs called retinoids—in almost all the cases I have seen, both proved to be ineffective as the lesions come back or simply emerge in another area. It is also not uncommon for there to be wound-healing disturbances in the scar area.

If patients with acne inversa are overweight, it is important to tell them that losing weight or wearing looser clothing may help avoid skin irritation. This type of acne also responds very well to dietary changes. Thus, it is also essential to inform those patients about which foods to avoid (see Chapter 8).

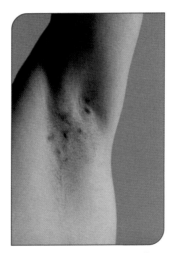

ACNE INVERSA–ARMPIT[5]

Acne Rosacea

Acne rosacea, usually referred to as rosacea, is often mistaken for acne vulgaris in its early stages. It is characterized by redness, papules, pustules, and swelling (of the nose). This condition is discussed in detail in Chapter 9, including characteristic differences between acne vulgaris and acne rosacea, and treatment according to TCM.

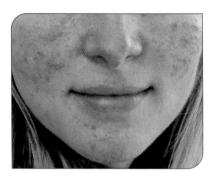 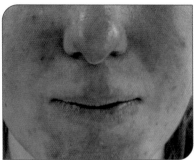

Current Treatment Options in Western Medicine
Topical Treatment

Depending on the type of acne, Western medicine usually recommends topical retinoids and anti-microbials for mild to moderate acne–in addition to special cosmetic treatments often offered by Western dermatologists, including skin-renewing exfoliation and special washes and skincare products. Retinoids are vitamin A acid derivatives. They fight pimples and blackheads, but do not help with a bacterial infection. Anti-microbial therapy comes in the form of antibiotic ointments and creams.

Systemic Treatment

For moderate to severe acne, the standard treatment in Western medicine is prescribing antibiotics topically and even orally, if the topical treatment has not been successful, in order to suppress *Propionibacterium acnes* (*P. acnes*). Systemic antibiotics act on the one hand by a reduction of the colonization of the sebaceous follicles by *P. acnes*, and on the other hand by a reduction of various pro-inflammatory mechanisms. Therefore, there is no linear dosage–response relationship. Plus, oral treatment with antibiotics needs time–results cannot be seen from one day to the next. Practice shows that for most medications the first signs of improvement in acne appear after six to eight weeks at the earliest, if at all.

Another option is the oral contraceptive pill. Acne is often attributed to hormonal changes–a seemingly easy fix for conventional medicine. Therefore, women are often prescribed the contraceptive pill for acne treatment.

Not all contraceptive pills are suitable for acne treatment (only those based on anti-androgens) and women clearly have to weigh the risks and benefits of this kind of treatment. For women who are trying to become pregnant, hormonal treatment is not an option. Some women are unable to take the contraceptive pill for medical reasons. And, of course, this is not a treatment option for male patients.

Possible Side Effects of Current Treatment Options in Western Medicine

Skin-renewing exfoliants can help with local acne treatment and they are mostly based on natural fruit acids, such as citric acid. The substance is applied to the affected skin, where it is allowed to act for a certain time. Exfoliation peels off the upper layers of the skin and prevents keratinization disorders of the skin. Exfoliation should be used with care and not too frequently as it stresses and irritates the skin. With fresh acne lesions and open skin lesions, I do not consider this aggressive form of treatment to be appropriate. Patients often confirm this perception as it can burn and is quite painful.

The treatment options Western medicine employs to tackle acne from within the body, however, are highly debatable at best and dangerous at worst. One option is antibiotics. This form of treatment is becoming less and less effective as there are more antibiotic-resistant strains of bacteria. In general, antibiotics are prescribed too often and too quickly.[6] We see this in daily practice or have perhaps already experienced it ourselves. Instead of only giving antibiotics when necessary, they are used like a sledgehammer for cracking a simple nut. And making bacteria increasingly resistant is not the only downside. Taken orally, the side effects of antibiotics are widely known. Many patients complain of gastrointestinal problems such as stomach pain and/or diarrhea while taking antibiotics and afterwards. Other common harmful side effects include allergies, skin rash, or nausea.[7] Applied topically, ointments and creams containing antibiotics change the pH value and the physiological amount of fat on the skin's surface. This should not be the general idea or purpose of any treatment. Many plants are known to have an anti-microbial action, so plant-based treatment seems to be an effective alternative to antibiotics.

The second treatment option is the contraceptive pill. However, there is a common misconception we need to address with patients. The pill is not a lifestyle drug and it shouldn't be taken just for skin conditions, including acne. In fact, it is unwise to use such a widespread form of treatment that interferes with the physiological processes of the body in such an extreme manner. It seems to be such an unhealthy approach to healing and we cannot want this for our patients. What is more, many patients report how bad they feel and that they want to come off the pill. Some might argue that patients' improved appearance outweighs the possible side effects of the pill. However, I would say that there is a reason that patients end up in our practice. Patients want a more natural approach that is effective and does not entail significant side effects. Every woman needs to make this decision for herself. She needs to be informed and weigh up the risks[8] and benefits of taking the pill. We should advise patients that the pill is not a treatment for anything! It does not regulate anything but only suppresses. If the pill is discontinued, the skin usually becomes as bad as before. Women know this and might not dare to stop this massive hormonal interference for this reason. And that cannot be the solution. In fact, many women come because they have previously had their skin flare up when stopping the pill, and they wish to pre-emptively address their skin before stopping the pill. This is where TCM comes in.

Endnotes

1   Tan, J.K.L. and Bhate, K. (2015) "A global perspective on the epidemiology of acne." *British Journal of Dermatology 172*, Suppl. 1, 3–12.

2   Schäfer, T., Nienhaus, A., Vieluf, D., Berger, J., and Ring J. (2001) "Epidemiology of acne in the general population: The risk of smoking." *British Journal of Dermatology 145*, 100–104.

3   Source: Shutterstock.

4   Comedones: non-inflammatory acne.

5   Source: Shutterstock.

6   Aslam, B., Wang, W., Arshad, M.I., Khurshid, M., *et al.* (2018) "Antibiotic resistance: A rundown of a global crisis." *Infection and Drug Resistance 11*, 1645–1658. doi:10.2147/IDR.S173867.

7   Smith, S.M., Fahey, T., Smucny, J., and Becker, L.A. (2014) "Antibiotics for acute bronchitis." *Cochrane Database of Systematic Reviews 1*, 3, CD000245. doi:10.1002/14651858.CD000245.pub3.

8   Sabatini, R., Cagiano, R., and Rabe, T. (2011) "Adverse effects of hormonal contraception." *Journal of Reproductive Medicine and Endocrinology 8*, Special issue 1, 130–156.

3

Overview and Basics of Chinese Dermatology

I T IS ASSUMED that the reader is familiar with the foundations of Traditional Chinese Medicine (TCM). This chapter on the basics of TCM dermatology is primarily aimed at TCM students and beginners. Experts can, of course, skip this chapter. Nonetheless, the information in this chapter can be a valuable resource and refresher for everyone–TCM dermatologists, general TCM doctors, and students of TCM.

An Overview of the History of Chinese Medical Dermatology (*pí fū kē* 皮肤科)

Chinese medical dermatology draws on many centuries of experience, with detailed records of the effects of Chinese herbs and acupuncture on the condition of the skin. Comprehensive descriptions of the treatment of specific skin diseases were put down in writing by ancient scholars, and their clinical histories and notes offer a depth of experience that we still utilize in our practice today.

Yet time does not stand still. A great deal of research into Chinese medicine has been conducted both inside and outside China. In addition to clinical studies, official monographs about almost every Chinese medical plant are available at the European Medicines Agency (EMEA) and the World Health Organization (WHO). These monographs provide a detailed introduction and scientific overview of the safety, efficacy, and quality control of commonly used medicinal plants in Chinese dermatology. Moreover, gathered information about chemical composition, pharmacological effects, toxicology, clinical studies, and research has been incorporated into many *materia medica*, the herbal textbooks used by TCM doctors worldwide.[1]

The result of this combination of a rich history and modern developments is an independent and sophisticated specialty in Chinese medicine, which can be effectively employed in the treatment of many, if not most, skin diseases. This is particularly true for the most common skin problems presenting in our clinics, where the effectiveness of conventional medicine therapy is often very poor.

Developmental Changes in Chinese Dermatology

In ancient China, Chinese dermatology was a part of the general category *wài kē* 外科. Medical fields such as traumatology and surgery were also classified as a part of *wài kē* at that time. *Wài* refers to the outside of the body and comprises the skin, hair, muscles, flesh, sinews, and bones. The term *kē* means subject, branch, or field. *Wài kē*, or "external medicine," refers to the diagnosis and treatment of conditions on the exterior of the body. This includes skin conditions such as sores and abscesses, and diseases of the eye, ear, nose, and mouth. In contrast, *nèi kē* 内科 (internal medicine) refers to diseases occurring inside the body and the *nèi*, or the inside, comprising the viscera and bowels. Chinese dermatology was recognized much later in history as a separate specialty in TCM.

The following presents a short overview on the development and documentation of Chinese dermatology.

Early classical literature	Small sections dedicated to Chinese dermatology (*pí fū kē*)	• Many important doctors devoted to the study and practice of external medicine • References to external medicine scattered in medical textbooks • No independent section of medical literature
Sòng Dynasty[2] 1263	*Wài Kē Jīng Yào* (Essence of Diagnosis and Treatment of External Diseases) by Chén Zì-Míng	• First book solely focused on *wài kē* • Establishment of external medicine and traumatic surgery as independent herbal branches of Chinese medicine
Yuán Dynasty[3] 1335	*Wài Kē Jīng Yì* (Treatment of Surgical Diseases) by Qí Dé-Zhī	• Compilation of the medical knowledge of external diseases prior to the Yuán Dynasty • Treatment of external diseases should start with regulating the body's internal system considering pathogenic factors • External disease arises from disharmony between yīn 阴 and yáng 阳, or stagnating qì 气 and *xuè* 血 • Creation of new therapies, e.g. wet compresses and methods for draining pus

Ming Dynasty[4]	Wāng Jī (1463–1539)	▪ Medical writer and clinical practitioner from Ānhuī Province south of Nánjīng
1531	*Wài Kē Lǐ Lì* (Exemplars for Applying the Principles of External Medicine)	▪ Preface: "external medicine [i.e. surgery] deals with ulcers, abscesses, sores and boils…seen on the exterior"
		▪ Wāng Jī's views on *wài kē*: "surgical" doctors (TCM dermatologists) do not perform the invasive surgery associated with surgeons today
		▪ All external manifestations of illness have internal roots
		▪ Emphasized the combination of internal treatments, i.e. herbal decoctions, and external treatments, i.e. ointments, washes, acupuncture, or moxibustion
		▪ Vast number of case histories
1522–1633	*Wāng Shíshān Yī Shū Bā Zhǒng* (Wāng Shíshān's Eight Medical Books)	▪ Numerous cases of *wài kē* categories, e.g. itchy body, foot sores, and breast lumps[5]
	One book of this compilation is *Shí Shān Yī Àn* (Medical Cases of Wāng Jī)	▪ More than one hundred of Wāng Jī's medical cases (collected by his students)
Ming and Qīng[6] Dynasties		▪ Chinese dermatology flourished with the publication of several works that presented treatment of external diseases
Late Ming Dynasty 1604	*Wài Kē Qǐ Xuán* (Profound Insights on External Diseases) by Shēn Dǒu-Yuán	▪ Consisting of 12 volumes
		▪ Considered China's first atlas of skin diseases
		▪ Contains about 200 different diseases and treatments
1617	*Wài Kē Zhèng Zōng* (True Lineage of External Medicine) by Chén Shí-Gōng	▪ New therapeutic recommendations for skin diseases, including ointments
		▪ Summary of medical achievements before the Ming Dynasty
		▪ Diagnoses, therapies, medical records, and prescriptions
		▪ Precise surgical procedures, e.g. removal of nasal polyps,[7] trachelorrhaphy, and cancer therapies
1665	*Wài Kē Dà Chéng* (Great Compendium of External Medicine) by Qí Kūn	▪ Chinese dermatology became increasingly sophisticated and numerous specialist books were published, such as the *Wài Kē Dà Chéng*

1740	*Wài Kē Zhèng Zhì Quán Shēng Jí* (Complete Compendium of Patterns and Treatments in External Medicine) by Wáng Wéi-Dé	▪ A summary of 40 years' clinical experience ▪ In the treatment of sores: division into yáng-type (red, excessive) and yīn-type (white, cold, qì and blood stagnation) pattern ▪ Treating yīn-type patterns by activating the yáng and supplementing qì and blood ▪ Many warming and blood stasis-dispelling formulas
1831	*Wài Kē Zhèng Zhì Quán Shū* (Complete Book of Patterns and Treatments in External Medicine) by Xǔ Kè-Chāng	▪ Based on the former book, similar academic thoughts ▪ Division of syndromes into two categories, namely those with definite location and those without a definite location ▪ Pointed out the importance of Stomach qì and opposed the abuse of cold and attacking medicines ▪ One volume includes different treatments on poisoning, e.g. food poisoning, animal poisoning, etc.

▪ Most classics on external diseases and treatments reprinted in modern times
▪ New dermatological textbooks
▪ Some available in English

The Daily Routine in Chinese Medical Dermatology

Dermatology is one of the most difficult areas of TCM. The disease patterns are complex and many skin diseases are deep-rooted and resistant to treatment. The challenge of diagnosing and treating skin diseases requires a highly skilled ability to observe and to analyze. Every student of Chinese medicine soon finds that the knowledge one acquires from one's teachers cannot simply be copied in clinic: imitation will not work; you must use your teacher's knowledge as a basis to build your own expertise. There are some factors that cannot be adapted, such as environmental circumstances or emotional and cultural factors. No matter how much experience you have gained throughout the years, the continuing process of learning from experienced teachers enables you to deepen both theoretical and practical understanding, learning refinements that improve your practice and prevent mistakes in application. This is the only way to deepen expertise and refine knowledge—an experience that will serve your patients as well.

A constant challenge in daily practice is that disease patterns often overlap. It is also important to note that most patients who come into a TCM practice have a long history of visiting allopathic skin specialists and have already tried multiple therapies. Again, most cases present not only with a skin disorder but also with other factors such as digestive or emotional issues. This is why patience is required from both the doctor and the patient over the course of the treatment. Patients need to be made aware of the fact that long-term conditions will take much longer to treat than conditions with a more recent onset.

Chinese dermatology deals with profound processes that manifest on the body's surface–the skin. Skin diseases must be understood in the context of the entire body, a perspective that is fundamentally different from conventional medicine. Diseases are considered through complex patterns of signs and symptoms that define each individual clinical presentation. In TCM, the goal is always to treat the pattern, which is regarded as the root cause. In other words, a purely symptom-based treatment as is frequently employed in conventional Western dermatology will not reach such a long-lasting resolution.

The initial diagnosis of the skin disease leaves us with multiple options for internal and external treatments. The following presents a step-by-step assessment of this process.

For a correct diagnosis of skin diseases according to TCM, it is essential to consider the following factors:

- an examination of the skin lesion (its onset, duration, location, appearance, and temperature)

- the exacerbating or relieving factors

- all associated symptoms such as itching, pain, burning sensation, scaling,[8] bleeding, or pus and discharge.

The focus in Chinese dermatology is always the skin lesion with all its presenting characteristics. Besides the presenting skin disease, factors such as emotions, sleep, diet, digestion, lifestyle (potential stress, overwork, night shifts), and environment, and the menstrual cycle in female patients, are important aspects of the Chinese diagnostic process. Moreover, by taking pulse and tongue diagnosis into consideration, the therapist gathers information on how the body works as a whole. Then, once the Chinese diagnosis has been established, an individual treatment plan is created.

In severe or long-lasting skin diseases, Chinese herbs can be prescribed for both internal treatment and external application. One issue is important but often overlooked: in stubborn cases, it is particularly important to enquire more closely about diet, living circumstances, and lifestyle habits. This is especially true for those patients with a chronic skin disease who expect instant results, or patients who state that they have already tried every method available. Practitioners might be surprised what they will learn about bad eating habits, excessive alcohol consumption, or a constant lack of sleep. For those patients, it is essential to provide dietary advice and to explain what role their own behavior plays in maintaining their disease. Telling them to go to bed early or to reduce their workload to lessen stress may seem to be simple and obvious advice, but patients often find it hard to break habits. One approach is to help the patient understand that they are doing it for themselves. If you can help a patient realize that they are a part of the therapeutic process, substantial progress can be made.

Chinese Herbal Treatment Options in Chinese Medical Dermatology

The wide variety of treatment options developed over the centuries and the extensive range of internal and external applications that TCM offers are a direct response to the flexibility required in curing complex disease patterns.

This section offers a general overview of commonly used internal and external treatment options in Chinese medical dermatology. Advantages and disadvantages of the available applications will be explained, and examples are listed by way of illustration. All of this is part of basic Chinese medicine education, but it can be helpful for explaining it to your patient and can serve as an overview for students and beginners. A brief outline of specific external treatment options for acne can be found in Appendix I.

Decoctions (*Jiān Jì* 煎剂)

Decoctions, or teas, of raw herbs are the most effective form of treatment. Herbal decoctions are prepared in three steps: first soaking, which allows the cell walls of the medicinal substances to expand for better extraction during boiling; then boiling in a ceramic pot (a ceramic pot is usually the best choice, because herbs such as *ē jiāo*, *hé shǒu wū*, or *shú dì huáng* are not suitable for cooking in a metal pot); and lastly straining. The patient then drinks the strained liquid. To obtain the highest efficacy of the herbs when brewing, the herbs are usually boiled twice. Some herbs are added early, some later; some herbs are bagged and others are dissolved in water and taken directly without boiling.

Each prescription combines individual medicinal herbs selected in each case to fulfill the individual's needs. Decoctions are flexible in their application and allow easy adaptation of the prescription to the condition as it presents on a particular day. Thus, the patient will obtain an individually tailored prescription fitting his or her medical condition and current situation. One single pill can never be effective for thousands of patients, as seen in conventional medicine, when every one of these people has their own individual symptoms and different situation in life.

The substances extracted from a freshly brewed herbal decoction are more potent than from other forms of prepared Chinese herbal medicine. Raw herbs can also be modified through processing techniques, known as *páo zhì* 炮制. *Páo zhì* is a traditional preparation process, which changes and specifies the therapeutic effect of medicinal plants. It reduces toxicity and unwanted side effects, changes pharmacological properties, enhances the precision of therapeutic effects, and changes the smell and taste of the plants. There are different preparation methods, such as roasting, frying, steaming, baking, calcining, germinating, fermenting, or cooking individually or in special combinations. Applied in daily practice, this means that if you want to change the action–for example, strengthen a certain effect of an herb–or you want to make it more tolerable for patients with a weak digestion, then you can use *páo zhì*–depending on your needs. Any qualified TCM pharmacist is able to prepare it.

Another advantage of herbal decoctions is that the ingredients can be cooked for different lengths of time. Flowers, for example, are very light in nature and should only be cooked for a few minutes. Heavy substances such as minerals should be cooked for a longer time, at least 60 minutes, and they are often pre-cooked for this reason. In general, a fresh herbal decoction with a long cooking time is best for deep-rooted processes because it can reach the deep layers of the body and quickly attack the disease. This means that the correct location of the disease must be taken into account in order to cure illness. For external applications, herbs are only very briefly boiled because the effects must address the surface.

In summary, within a complex and individual tailored herbal formula, many chemical reactions occur between the active ingredients of each single herb. The dosages of decoctions can be used with precision. A decoction can be modified in many ways and works fast. Additionally, in the West raw herbs are considerably cheaper than other application forms such as herbal granules. Considering all this, when treating a serious case, raw herbs are always recommended. Although herbal decoctions do not taste good, patients usually tolerate them once the benefits are explained. Herbal decoctions are usually the best choice to treat difficult skin conditions.

Granules (*Kē Lì Jì* 颗粒剂) and Pills (*Piàn Jì* 片剂)

Granules are Chinese medicinal herbs extracted and concentrated into granules, using modern extraction and concentration technologies to replicate the traditional method of preparing medicinal decoctions. In pills, the extracts are further processed and pressed into pill form for ease of consumption.

As granules and pills are not given in a fresh form, fillers such as cellulose and carrier substances such as lactose are added. Although there are no significant pharmacological, toxicological, and clinical studies to demonstrate equivalence with decoctions,[9] it can be seen in clinical practice that granules are less effective as symptoms return and conditions worsen when patients switch to granules. Moreover, it seems quite difficult to determine the exact ratio of herb available in the granules. The industry mentions several yield ratios–that is, the amount of product yielded from the extraction process. The standard yield ratio seems to be 5:1,[10] but the industry often does not publish the exact ratio because yields can differ. Factors such as whether the herbs (especially roots and fruits/seeds) are ground into smaller pieces, the length of extraction time, the solubility of the herb's ingredients in water, whether organic solvents are used, the pH of the extract solution, whether a temperature gradient is used, and the seasonality of the herb can all influence the final yield.[11] The size of the measuring spoon[12] used by patients and whether it is a level or heaped spoonful must also be taken into account. As a consequence of all of these factors, determining how to properly dose granules can be a very difficult process. Furthermore, for granules neither *páo zhì* nor different cooking time options are available. Simple practical disadvantages of granules are that they often clump together, they do not taste better than herbal decoctions, and they are usually more expensive than raw herbs.

However, granules are convenient and helpful in some situations, and better than no remedy–for instance, during travel, in circumstances where refrigeration is not available, or in situations where the patient does not want to or cannot drink decoctions, such as during pregnancy or after having taken decoctions for a long time. I find that many patients return after taking granules during travel and ask for herbal decoctions once more.

Tinctures (*Dīng Jì* 酊剂)

Tinctures are herbal preparations made in alcoholic bases. Tinctures are called medicinal liquor in Chinese, and they can be used internally or applied topically. Taken internally, the use of herbal tinctures is not common, but it can be a good interim solution when the patient is not drinking herbal tea. For example, patients are commonly advised to drink one bag of Chinese herbal tea per week in less severe conditions. One bag of tea does not usually last the whole week, and so for the remaining days of the week the patient should take the tincture to support the effect of the raw herbs. However, the use of tinctures for acne–externally and internally–is extremely rare.

Washes (*Xǐ Dí* 洗涤) and Wet Compresses (*Shī Fū* 湿敷)

Herbal washes, which are applied topically directly to the skin lesion, can help with various types of skin problems such as itching, heat, inflammation, pustules, swellings, and ulcerations, and promote healing of the skin. Herbal washes can be used as an external wash or as local wet compresses. For wet compresses, a folded piece of material, bandage, or small towel is immersed in herbal decoction and then placed over the affected area for a certain period of time. In general, herbal washes or wet compresses and also baths are mainly used in skin conditions that involve discharge. This method still allows the secretion of pathogenic fluids and pus while relieving heat, inflammation, pustules, or swellings. During acute stages of serious skin conditions, washes, compresses, and baths in particular should be taken with caution because of the potential risk of secondary inflammation.

Special herbal combinations are known to have a disinfecting effect, such as *Sān Huáng Xǐ Jì*, made of *huáng bǎi*, *huáng qín*, *dà huáng*, and *kǔ shēn*. Because "yellow" (*huáng* in Chinese) is part of three of these four herb names, the formula is called "Three Yellow Cleanser Formula." This ancient topical formula is known for its effects of clearing heat, stopping itching, and arresting secretion, and it is often used in skin conditions such as acne, dermatitis, eczema, and furuncles (boils). One other example for a very simple herbal wash, which is very often prescribed for acne relief, is wash consisting only of *zhāng nǎo* (camphor). We have seen this wash have very good results for relieving pain, swelling, and irritation in deep and painful pimples. But it has to be used with caution because *zhāng nǎo* is suitable for external application only. Patients should be informed that it is toxic if taken internally![13]

In summary, since the light texture of herbal decoctions offers a non-occluding effect when applied externally, this method is able to heal the skin on a deeper level. A cream, on the other hand, would enclose the discharge, and instead of pathogens exiting the body, they are trapped and move transversely back into the body. Interestingly, this is very often seen in conventional medicine. Although skin lesions are still discharging, patients are prescribed creams. The skin cannot breathe, the secretion or pus is trapped, and the healing process is thus impeded. The feedback of almost all patients is that they intuitively do not feel comfortable with creams when the wound is still weeping.

Pastes (*Hú Jì* 糊剂)

Pastes are prepared by combining finely powdered herbs with a carrier substance. One type of paste is prepared using a greasy medium such as oil. In Chinese dermatology, sesame oil is very frequently used. The other type of paste is prepared with water. The paste is then applied to the affected area of the skin in order to protect dry skin, serve as a barrier, protect the affected area from bacterial infection, and promote the healing process of the skin.

Pastes should not be applied topically if there is profuse discharge. They should also be avoided in case of damp-heat (*shī rè* 湿热), as damp-heat could move transversely back inside to the interior and the pathogenic process would be aggravated. Zōu Yuè pointed out in his *Wài Kē Zhēn Quán* (Personal Experience in *Wài Kē*, 1838) that "pastes are contraindicated when damp-heat toxins exist on the lower extremities. If misused, the confined heat will move transversely and spread even more extensively. Pastes are advisable in protected cases." Therefore, the application of pastes when the patient shows profuse pus or discharge will impede the drainage of the fluids.[14]

A very commonly used paste is *Jīn Huáng Sǎn* (Golden Yellow Powder)[15] mixed with an oil base. This paste is applied to a wide range of disorders in dermatology and trauma. It clears heat, removes toxins, dispels dampness, eliminates blood stasis, and reduces swelling. It is thus very useful for inflammation, swellings, and pain in skin conditions such as acne, carbuncles, and insect bites.

Ointments (*Yóu Gāo* 油膏)

An ointment, also called a salve or balm, is a semi-solid preparation for external application on damaged skin. Oil-based ointments consist of finely powdered herbs heated in an oil base, such as almond oil, jojoba oil, or sesame oil. Sesame seeds are known to have the highest oil content. Sesame oil can be extracted from normal seeds or seeds that have been roasted prior to being processed. The oil of roasted sesame seeds is dark and smoky red, and has a distinctive aroma produced from the toasting and crushing of the seeds. This toasted sesame oil, often used in Chinese cooking, is particularly suitable for making oil-based ointments because it is comparatively stable and does not turn rancid on contact with air due to the toasting process. The texture of an oil-based ointment is thick and often looks yellowish. Creams, by contrast, are water-soluble and usually have a white hue. An ointment can be smoothly applied on damaged skin and it is absorbed easily and quickly. Ointments usually have good permeability and are therefore often used after herbal baths and washes.

Oil-based ointments are often used to stop itching, clear heat, and dispel inflammation. Ointments are particularly suitable for chronic skin diseases or when the skin is very thick, such as seen in neurodermatitis. Ointments, like pastes, are contraindicated if there is profuse discharge.

Creams (*Rǔ Gāo* 乳膏)

A cream is a semi-solid emulsion of either oil in water or water in oil for topical use. Creams are spreadable substances, similar to ointments but not as thick, and they seem to be more appropriate for application on exposed skin areas such as the face and hands.

For compound creams, either oil-based herbal extracts or water-based herbal extracts (decoctions) are carefully blended with the base cream and other substances such as essential oils, aloe vera, or dexpanthenol[16] to achieve a homogenous and consistent product. In Chinese dermatology, base creams often consist of high-quality and skin-friendly substances such as shea butter, cocoa butter, jojoba oil, or natural white beeswax. It should be emphasized that petroleum jelly (e.g. Vaseline®) should not be used, although it is still often mentioned in medical textbooks. Petroleum jelly, a petroleum by-product of the oil industry, is not a high-quality solution. It is thick and often poorly spreadable, and has an unpleasant smell. Cheap and low-quality substances such as petroleum jelly, paraffin, or propylene glycol usually leave a greasy film on the skin with increased sweating underneath. In sweating, salt crystals are produced, which can further worsen already existing itching, and therefore these substances should be avoided. For those who still prefer to use petroleum jelly, wool wax alcoholic cream (also called lanolin) can be used as an alternative. Wool wax alcoholic cream is a cream base, consisting of white petroleum jelly, cetyl-stearyl alcohol, and wool wax alcohol. Due to its lighter texture, it spreads easily and feels more pleasant on the skin.

However, when making your own creams and ointments, it is important to know exactly what ingredients are being used. Only pure, natural, environmentally friendly options should be used, ensuring that the ingredients do not irritate the skin and are suitable for sensitive skincare. If there is an ingredient a patient is allergic to, one can simply leave it out or replace it with something else.

One instance in daily practice in which creams are frequently used is neurodermatitis. In neurodermatitis, lichenification can be seen; the skin is usually very dry, with scaling and itching. The patient feels very uncomfortable: as well as the visual appearance and itching sensation, the skin feels very tight. This is often quite painful. In this case, creams made from herbs such as *shēng dì huáng, dāng guī, gān cǎo, sāng shèn,* or *bǎi hé* are frequently prescribed. Another common instance in daily practice in which creams are frequently used is psoriasis. In this case, a simple cream consisting of just one herb, *qīng dài,* is proven to be very effective—*Qīng Dài Gāo* (Indigo Cream). It can clear heat, resolve toxicity, cool blood, reduce swelling, and inhibit the growth of cells. It should be mentioned, however, that these kinds of creams should be prescribed only when the skin has healed and skin fissures are closed.

In order to treat the root cause of the disease, internal TCM remedies must be at the center of treatment. Nonetheless, external applications are often also prescribed. According to clinical experience, external treatments supplement and enhance the healing process, and the effect for the patient is more immediate. And we cannot underestimate the psychological factor here. The patient is more directly involved in the application of external remedies and thus can participate actively. This can be very important for some patients.

One more practical hint: patients themselves are quite often very sensitive and easily have an allergic reaction to various kinds of external influences. Some patients say that they are even sensitive to water. This is why it is always advisable to start with a mild approach when it comes to external treatments.

Endnotes

1 For example, Bensky, D., Clavey, S., and Stöger, E. (2004) *Materia Medica,* 3rd edition. Seattle, WA: Eastland Press; Chen, J.K. (2013) *Chinese Medical Herbology and Pharmacology.* City of Industry, CA: Art of Medicine Press.

2 Sòng Dynasty: Běi Sòng, Nán Sòng (Northern Sòng, Southern Sòng) (960–1279 AD).

3 Yuán Dynasty (1206–1368 AD).

4 Míng Dynasty (1368–1644 AD).

5 Grant, J. (2003) *A Chinese Physician: Wang Ji and the Stone Mountain Medical Case Histories.* Abingdon: Routledge.

6 Qīng Dynasty (before the Opium Wars of 1840) (1644–1911/12 AD).

7   With a pair of copper wires and a loop at the end of each wire.

8   Scaling is very rarely seen in acne.

9   Luo, H., Li, Q., Flower, A., Lewith, G., and Liu, J. (2012) "Comparison of effectiveness and safety between granules and decoction of Chinese herbal medicine: A systematic review of randomized clinical trials." *Journal of Ethnopharmacology 140*, 3, 555–567.

10 Sturgeon, S. (2012) *Powders and Granules RCHM*. Norwich: Register of Chinese Herbal Medicine.

11 Sturgeon, S. (2011) "Questions and Answers about Extract Powders/ Granules–Part One." *The Mayway Mailer*, November 2011. Accessed on 1/21/2021 at www.mayway.com/pdfs/maywaymailers/Skye-Sturgeon-QM-Extract-powder-11-2011.pdf.

12 Teaspoon, tablespoon, etc.

13 *Zhāng nǎo* will be discussed in more detail in Appendix I.

14 Taken from my TCM Dermatology seminar notes.

15 *Jīn Huáng Sǎn: huáng bǎi, dà huáng, jiāng huáng, bái zhǐ, hòu pò, chén pí, cāng zhú, tiān nán xīng, gān cǎo.*

16 Dexpanthenol, also known as panthenol, pantothenol, or provitamin B5, is often used as a moisturizer and to improve wound healing in creams, ointments, and lotions.

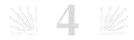

The Traditional Chinese Medicine Perspective on Acne

The History of Acne According to Traditional Chinese Medicine

Like many other diseases, acne has been treated with Chinese medicine for a very long time. Throughout the last two thousand years, from the early Qín to the late Qīng Dynasty, doctors explored and summarized their knowledge gained through long-term clinical observation and practice. The wealth of experience is therefore of great magnitude. TCM syndrome differentiation and understanding of the pathogenesis of acne has always been, and continues to be, refined and improved. Every day, we rely on this ancient knowledge in our practices, which helps us give our patients the best possible treatment. However, every TCM doctor should feel free to incorporate their own experiences in the treatment of acne patients. The treatment has to be adapted to many different circumstances. Hence, doctors also have to learn to be flexible.

Before we delve into detailed TCM syndrome differentiation, we will first take a look at the history of acne according to TCM in order to understand the development and changes in the treatment of this skin condition.

The Definition and History of Acne According to Traditional Chinese Medicine

Every culture and every generation has its own approach towards health– and life in general. The language of such a culture changes constantly, as does all language. Therefore, it is no surprise that the understanding, treatment methods, and terminology for acne[1] has varied over time. Many different names can be found in ancient texts when describing acne, but today TCM refers to acne as *fèi fēng fěn cì* 肺风粉刺, also called "Lung-wind acne," "lesion of Lung wind," or "Lung-wind white thorns"–or, in short, "*fěn cì*" (acne). The name *fèi fēng fěn cì* is derived from the shape of the eruptions on the face, which look like rice grains or thorns (*cì* 刺) and its connection to the Lung (*fèi* 肺) and the invasion of wind (*fēng* 风).

According to TCM theory, the skin is closely related to the Lungs as they control the skin by spreading (diffusing) fluids towards the skin and into the space between the skin and the muscles. The Lungs receive these fluids from the Spleen. If this diffusion mechanism functions as it should, the skin is nourished and moistened, and looks lustrous and healthy. An impairment of this function leads to malnourishment and dehydration of the skin. The Lungs are also in charge of controlling the opening and closing of the pores. In a healthy state, the opening and closing of the pores is well regulated, sweating will be normal, and the person is resilient. If the function of the Lungs is impaired, the space between the skin and the muscles may be too open, in which case a person sweats too much and pathogenic factors from outside can penetrate the body easily. The body's defenses drop and the person easily gets sick. The other option is that the pores are too tight. In this case, sweat cannot go out and pathogenic factors that have already invaded the body will usually cause strong reactions, such as high fever. All this shows how important the Lungs are for a healthy skin and immune defense.

As mentioned above, the understanding and description of acne has changed over time. The following lists an overview of acne and how it is described in classical TCM books and sources.[2]

| Qín and Hàn Dynasties (221–206 BC) (206 BC–220 AD)[3] | *Huáng Dì Nèi Jīng* (The Yellow Emperor's Inner Classic), author unknown | ▪ Earliest reference to the term "*cuó*" 痤[4] ▪ Earliest ancient description of acne as disease, its cause, and pathogenesis ▪ Pathogenesis: wind (*fēng* 风) attacks the body after sweating, and Lung qì (*fèi qì* 肺气) is constrained inside ▪ Points out that acne can be caused by dampness (*shī* 湿) attacking the skin when the interstitial space[5] is loose, and sweat pores are open after sweating |

Qín and Hàn Dynasties (221–206 BC) (206 BC–220 AD)	*Yǎng Shēng Fāng* (Formulas for Nourishing Life), author unknown	• Cause of acne: drinking alcohol[6] generates heat (*rè* 热), heat can move upwards up attacking the face • Combination of heat[7] and cold water[8] can cause acne
Eastern Jìn Dynasty (317–420)	*Zhǒu Hòu Bèi Jí Fāng* (Emergency Formulas to Keep Up One's Sleeve) by Gě Hóng	• First recorded prescription for treating acne • Cause of acne: young people are full of vigor and vitality
Northern and Southern Dynasties (420–589)	*Shén Nóng Běn Cǎo Jīng Jí Zhù* (Collected Commentaries on Shén Nóng's Materia Medica) by Táo Hóng-Jīng	• Earliest recorded medical book of TCM for treating acne • First mention of two herbs for treating acne: "*zǐ cǎo*" and "*shān zhū yú*"
Suí Dynasty (589–618)	*Zhū Bìng Yuán Hòu Lùn* (General Treatise on the Etiology and Symptomology of Diseases) by Cháo Yuán-Fāng	• Alcohol as important cause of acne • Acne occurs when the body is attacked by wind after drinking alcohol, or washing the face with cold water after alcohol consumption • Acne is described as "*miàn pào*" 面疱, a kind of face blister (pimples), which is caused by wind-heat (*fēng rè* 风热) • Acne is also described as "*sì miàn*" 嗣面, when it is caused by accumulation of wind and body fluids (*jīn yè* 津液)—pimples with white heads, like millet
Táng Dynasty (618–907)	*Zhù Shì Huáng Dì Nèi Jīng Sù Wèn* (Annotations on The Yellow Emperor's Inner Classic) by Wáng Bīng	• Location of acne: in the interstitial space, which is superficial • Thus, best treat with exterior-releasing method • Pathogenesis: yáng qì 阳气 is constrained inside the body and blood (*xuè* 血) and pus (*nóng* 脓) cannot be exuded
Táng Dynasty (618–907)	*Qiān Jīn Yì Fāng* (Supplement to Important Formulas Worth a Thousand Gold Pieces) by Sūn Sī-Miǎo	• Mentions various treatments–from simple treatment of acne to the treatment of acne scars
Sòng Dynasty (960–1279)	*Tài Píng Shèng Huì Fāng* (Taiping Holy Prescriptions for Universal Relief) by Wáng Huái-Yín	• Deficiency as root cause of acne • Wind and body fluids can accumulate in the skin

Sòng Dynasty (960–1279)	*Shèng Jì Zōng Lù* (Comprehensive Recording of Sacred Relief) by Northern Sòng Government (Physicians of the Sòng Imperial Court)	▪ Heat in the Lung meridian steams the Lung, causing heat accumulation in the skin
Míng Dynasty (1368–1644)	*Gǔ Jīn Yī Tǒng Dà Quán* (The Complete Compendium of Ancient and Modern Medical Works) by Xú Chūn-Fǔ	▪ Acne is named "*fēng cì*" 风刺 ▪ Cause of acne: yáng is obstructed by yīn
Míng Dynasty (1368–1644)	*Yī Xué Gāng Mù* (The Grand Compendium of Medicine) by Lóu Yīng	▪ Constitutional deficiency as root of acne ▪ Sweating, invasion of wind
Míng Dynasty (1368–1644)	*Wàn Bìng Huí Chūn* (The Restoration of Health from the Myriad Diseases) by Gǒng Tíng-Xián	▪ Yīn deficiency and frenetic stirring of ministerial fire can cause acne
Míng Dynasty (1368–1644)	*Shòu Shì Bǎo Yuán* (Prolonging Life and Preserving the Origin) by Gǒng Tíng-Xián	▪ Lung heat as root cause of acne
Míng Dynasty (1368–1644)	*Wài Kē Zhèng Zōng* (True Lineage of External Medicine) by Chén Shí-Gōng	▪ Acne is a kind of Lung disease ▪ Blood heat (*xuè rè* 血热) constraint in the Lung as cause of acne
Qīng Dynasty (1644–1911/12)	*Dòng Tiān Ào Zhǐ* (Secrets of External Medicine) by Chén Shì-Duó	▪ Causes of acne: wind-heat in Lung, wind-cold attacking the face, blood-heat (*xuè rè* 血热), damp-heat (*shī rè* 湿热), blood stasis (*xuè yū* 血瘀), etc.
Qīng Dynasty (1644–1911/12)	*Yī Jīng Yuán Zhǐ* (The Original Meaning of Medical Classics) by Xuē Xuě	▪ Pathogenesis of acne: insecurity of yáng qì
Qīng Dynasty (1644–1911/12)	*Zhēn Jiǔ Féng Yuán* (Encountering the Sources of Acupuncture and Moxibustion) by Lǐ Xué-Chuān	▪ Acne and tumor[9] are of the same kind but different in severity[10] ▪ Their difference lies in depth and degree
Qīng Dynasty (1644–1911/12)	*Yī Zōng Jīn Jiàn* (The Golden Mirror of Ancestral Medicine) by Wú Qiān *et al.*	▪ Blood heat in the Lung meridian as cause of acne
The Republic of China (1912–1949)	*Mài Jué Xīn Biān* (New Version of Pulse Diagnosis) by Liú Běn-Chāng	▪ Too much speaking hurts the Lung qì, resulting in weakness ▪ Drinking alcohol leads to damp-heat

The History of Treatment of Acne According to Traditional Chinese Medicine

The following table explains what kinds of treatments were applied at different time periods.[11] Interestingly, many of the herbs and formulas are still used today, which speaks for their effectiveness. Acupuncture plays an insignificant role in the treatment of acne in these old books. There are virtually no indications to be found in the source texts, whereas herbal prescriptions and individual herbs are described in detail for internal and external application (for washes and powders).

Eastern Jìn Dynasty (317–420)		
Zhǒu Hòu Bèi Jí Fāng (Emergency Formulas to Keep Up One's Sleeve) by Gě Hóng	*Pào Chuāng Fāng* (Blister and Sore Formula)	*huáng lián,*[12] *mǔ lì* • Grind the herbs into a fine powder and mix them with water • Apply the paste topically on the affected skin lesions Use: an effective formula for treating sores (*chuāng* 疮)[13]
	Dōng Kuí Sǎn (Cluster Mallow Fruit Powder)	*dōng kuí zǐ, bǎi zǐ rén, dōng guā zǐ, fú líng* • Grind the herbs into a fine powder • For internal use Use: can whiten the face[14]
Táng Dynasty (618–907)		
Qiān Jīn Yì Fāng (Supplement to Important Formulas Worth a Thousand Gold Pieces) by Sūn Sī-Miǎo	*Zhì Miàn Zhā Fāng* (Treating Facial Sore)	*mù lán pí*[15] • Marinate *mù lán pí* with vinegar for three years and dry it • Grind the dried herb into a fine powder and take it with warm wine Use: for treating facial sores
	Zhì Miàn Pào Fāng (Facial Acne Treatment)	*mù lán pí, zhī zǐ* • Grind the herbs into a fine powder, mix them together with honey, and apply as a facial mask to the skin Use: for treating facial sores
Wài Tái Mì Yào (Arcane Essentials from the Imperial Library) by Wáng Tāo	*Mù Lán Gāo Fāng* (Blond Magnolia Cream–Mu Lan Cream)	*mù lán pí, fáng fēng, bái zhǐ, qīng mù xiāng, niú xī, dú huó, gǎo běn, sháo yào, bái fù zǐ, dù héng,*[16] *dāng guī, xì xīn, chuān xiōng, shè xiāng* • Grind the herbs except *shè xiāng* • Fry them with pork oil three times • Discard the dregs and mix the herbs with *shè xiāng* • For external use Use: for treating facial sores

Sòng Dynasty (960–1279)

Tài Píng Shèng Huì Fāng (Taiping Holy Prescriptions for Universal Relief) by Wáng Huái-Yǐn	*Zhì Fěn Cì Jí Miàn Chuāng Fāng* (Acne and Facial Sore Formula)	*huáng lián, jīng mǐ, chì xiǎo dòu, wú zhū yú, shuǐ yín*[17] ■ Grind the herbs and mix them with sesame oil to form an adhesive paste ■ For external use Use: for treating acne and facial sores
	Zhì Miàn Shàng Pào Zǐ Fāng (Facial Blister Formula)	*dà huáng* ■ Grind the herb into a fine powder ■ Mix it with water to form an adhesive paste ■ For external use Use: for treating facial sores
Shèng Jì Zǒng Lù (Comprehensive Recording of Sacred Relief) by Northern Sòng Government (Physicians of the Sòng Imperial Court)	*Bái Liǎn Gāo Tú Fāng* (Ampelopsis Root Cream)	*bái liǎn,*[18] *bái shí zhī, xìng rén* ■ Grind the herbs and mix them with egg white for external use ■ Apply before going to bed Use: for treating facial sores
	Xuān Cǎo Gāo Tú Fāng (Day Lily Cream)	*xuān cǎo huā* (dried) ■ Grind the flower and mix it with honey ■ For external use after washing the face Use: for treating facial sores

Jīn Dynasty (1115–1234)

Sù Wèn Bìng Jī Qì Yí Bǎo Mìng Jí (Collection of Writings on the Mechanism of Disease, Suitability of Qì, and the Safeguarding of Life as Discussed in the "Basic Questions") by Liú Wán-Sù	*Fáng Fēng Tōng Shèng Sǎn* (Ledebouriella Sage-Inspired Powder)	*fáng fēng, sháo yào, dāng guī, chuān xiōng, dà huáng, máng xiāo, huáng qí, bái zhú, zhī zǐ, jīng jiè, shēng jiāng, shí gāo, jié gěng, huá shí, gān cǎo, lián qiào, bò hé, má huáng* ■ Mix all herbs and grind them into a fine powder ■ For internal use Treatment principle: dispel wind in the interstitial space; harmonize *yíng* 营 (nutritive) and *wèi* 卫 (defense)

Míng Dynasty (1368–1644)		
Wàn Bìng Huí Chūn (The Restoration of Health from the Myriad Diseases) by Gŏng Tíng-Xián	*Liù Wèi Dì Huáng Wán* (Six Ingredient Pill with Rehmannia)	*shú dì, shān yào, shān zhū yú, fú líng, zé xiè, mǔ dān pí* ▪ Mix and decoct raw herbs ▪ For internal use Treatment principle: treats the pattern of vigorous fire due to yīn deficiency
	Qīng Fèi Săn (Clear the Lungs Powder)	*lián qiáo, chuān xiōng, bái zhĭ, huáng lián, kŭ shēn, jīng jiè, sāng bái pí, huáng qín, zhī zĭ, zhè bèi mŭ, gān căo* ▪ Mix all herbs and grind them into a fine powder ▪ For internal use Treatment principle: clears heat from the Lungs; drains fire
Shòu Shì Băo Yuán (Prolonging Life and Preserving the Origin) by Gŏng Tíng-Xián	*Shēng Má Bái Zhĭ Tāng* (Rhizoma Cimicifugae and Radix Angelicae Dahuricae Decoction)	*shēng má, bái zhĭ, gān căo, cāng zhú, rén shēn, gé gēn, huáng qí, gān căo* ▪ Mix and decoct raw herbs ▪ For internal use Treatment: best taken in the morning so yáng qì can ascend to the face
Wài Kē Zhèng Zōng (True Lineage of External Medicine) by Chén Shí-Gōng	*Yù Jī Săn* (Jade Skin Powder)	*lǜ dòu, huá shí, bái zhĭ, bái fù zī* ▪ Grind the herbs into a fine powder and mix it with water ▪ For external use, after washing the face Use: treats facial acne with itching
Qīng Dynasty (1644–1911/12)		
Wài Kē Dà Chéng (Great Compendium of External Medicine) by Qí Kūn	*Pí Pá Qīng Fèi Yĭn* (Eriobotrya Decoction to Clear the Lung)[19]	*pí pá yè, sāng bái pí, huáng lián, huáng băi, rén shēn, gān căo* ▪ Mix and decoct raw herbs ▪ For internal use The earliest citation of this formula; still used quite frequently in contemporary practice

Differentiation of Acne According to the Affected Areas

Acne mostly occurs on the face, mainly on the forehead, cheeks, chin, and around the mouth, but it also can affect the chest (décolletage), back, upper arms, and shoulders. It can be restricted to one location or appear in multiple locations at the same time. An occurrence of acne lesions in the face and on the back is not uncommon; in fact, it happens very often.

Forehead

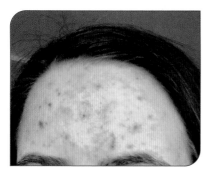
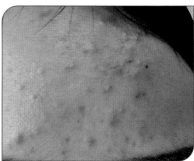

Temples

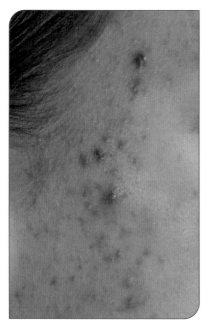
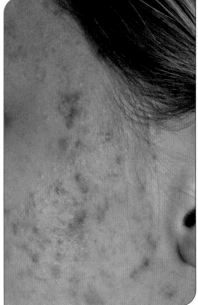

Cheeks

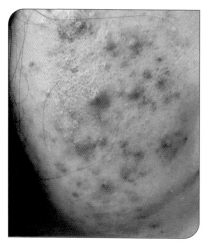
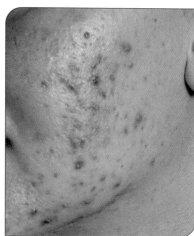

Chin

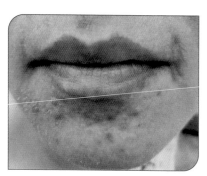
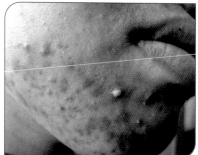

Around the Mouth

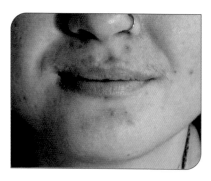
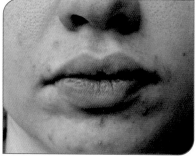

Chest

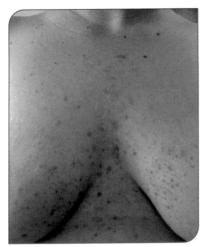
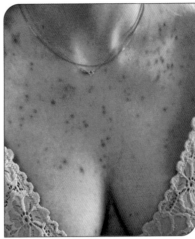

Back

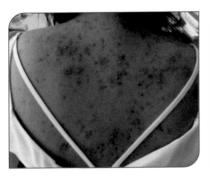
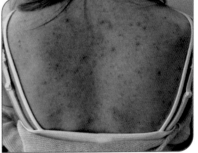

Arms and Shoulders

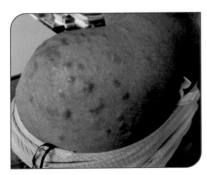
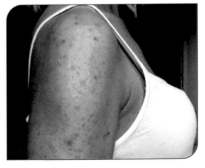

Face Mapping

Depending on where the acne appears, we may draw conclusions about the affected organ according to TCM. Of course, other symptoms and tongue and pulse diagnoses must also be taken into account. However, face mapping can be a telling factor and may help further questioning.

Face mapping is a basic concept, which helps identify the root cause of skin conditions such as acne by dividing the face into "zones." These different zones are connected to specific organs, and therefore skin irregularities in these zones indicate possible internal and organic imbalances and/or disorders that trigger the patient's skin condition. Face mapping is simply based on the construct and understanding that everything on the outside–that is, our skin–directly reflects our insides.[20] After all, our organs–and this includes the skin–are all connected through the meridians. In face mapping, we regard the face as a microcosm reflecting the entire body. And as each part of the face has a distinct relationship with an internal organ, this method guides us in determining the internal workings of the body.

There are several quite different approaches in the literature regarding face mapping. However, I have found the *Sù Wèn* to be a good and helpful starting point. The *Sù Wèn Cì Rè* (素问·刺热)[21] says:

> In the case of heat disease in the Liver, the left cheek becomes red first.
>> In the case of heat disease in the Heart, the forehead becomes red first.
>> In the case of heat disease in the Spleen, the nose becomes red first.
>> In the case of heat disease in the Lung, the right cheek becomes red first.
>> In the case of heat disease in the Kidneys, the chin becomes red first.

This book continues to explain the zones, which helps us make the mapping more distinct:

- Liver: "The cheek is the lower region in front of the ears." "If one stands upright facing the south, then it is his left cheek."

- Heart: "顏[22] is the section above the two eyebrows up to the frontal hairline. It is commonly called 額頭.[23]"

- Spleen: "The spleen qì is associated with the soil. The soil flourishes in the centre. The nose is located in the centre of the face. Hence [the spleen qì] manifests itself through the nose."

- Lung: "The lung [is] metal [and] is located on the right. Hence in the case of a heat disease in the lung, the right cheek is red first."

- Kidneys: "The kidney qì is associated with water. Water moistens only that which is below; it produces clear signs. Hence its signs appear at the chin."

This ancient theory clearly details the zones in the face. The illustration below represents the facial zones I have learned from my teachers. It is simple and quick, so quite suitable for our work in practice. I find this helpful as an additional indicator when treating patients with acne. Please keep in mind, however, that there are no clear lines determining the facial zones. The clinical signs are certainly more important, but the areas in the face may serve as a first indicator and often show the direction in which further questions should lead.

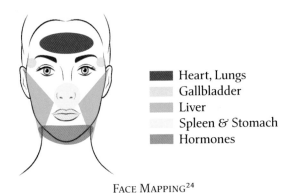

Heart, Lungs
Gallbladder
Liver
Spleen & Stomach
Hormones

FACE MAPPING[24]

- Forehead: The forehead is linked to the Heart, the Lungs, and respiratory system. You may ask your patient about possible mental stress, high blood pressure, poor circulation, allergies, asthma, or smoking, to name just a few factors.

- Temples: The corners of the forehead, the temples, are associated with the Gallbladder. The Gallbladder has a very close relationship to the Liver. Supressed emotions, excess anger, and stress will not just affect the Liver but also the partner organ, the Gallbladder. It can also make sense to ask the patient about their eating habits. The Gallbladder does not like greasy, fatty, and spicy foods, or alcohol, which also applies to the Liver, of course. Patients should be informed how important it is to have a healthy and balanced diet in order to have clear skin.

- Cheeks: Breakouts on the cheeks indicate a problem with the Liver. According to TCM, each organ system has a corresponding emotion, and for the Liver it is anger. You should pay close attention to whether your patient is chronically angry and frustrated–please never underestimate the negative effects of suppressed emotions. They harm the body just as much as more obvious and clearly visible emotions. In practice, we often see that this region stretches to the jaw. Therefore, "cheek" does not refer to the area surrounding the cheek bone towards the nose, but rather the outer part from the cheek bone along the ear to the jawbone right up to the neck.

- Nose: The region around the nose relates to the digestive system (Spleen and Stomach). If the patient repeatedly has pimples in the nasal area, then you should definitely ask about the digestion and dietary habits. In the broadest sense, the area belonging to the digestive system can also be extended to the area around the mouth. Clinical practice has shown that patients with poor eating habits often have pimples around the mouth.

- Chin and lower jawline: Acne around the chin and lower jaw is linked to hormonal disturbances. In women, this can be seen when acne worsens in the days prior to menstruation, possibly also caused by stress. Working on the menstrual cycle either with Chinese herbs or acupuncture, for example, might be a good idea. It may also be useful to ask about stress and pressure, in combination with suggestions about how to reduce it.

Another practical hint: What I have often observed in practice is the connection between strong emotions and pimples in the chest area (décolletage). Therefore, if your patient does not mention emotional upheaval but you see acne in this area, it is worthwhile to ask carefully about emotional issues. Many patients then talk about relationship problems. I have certainly seen this: Sorrow in the heart negatively impacts the skin around the heart area.

All in all, face mapping serves as a guide and initial indicator. However, syndrome differentiation cannot be waived under any circumstances because, ultimately, the patient is treated according to the underlying TCM pattern.

Etiology and Pathogenesis of Acne According to Traditional Chinese Medicine

Acne can arise from several causes and, as we see in our practices, is usually due to a combination of several factors. In order to find the best TCM therapy, a holistic approach to the patient's symptoms is essential. For this, we need to assess their living situation, psycho-emotional factors, and their lifestyle habits. This will allow us to determine the root causes of acne, to distinguish between the different TCM syndromes and finally to select the appropriate formulas accordingly.

Psycho-Emotional Factors, the Effects on the *Zàng Fǔ* Organs, and Their Relation to Acne

Many instances show us that the soul and body are connected–that both emotional and physical situations factor into a complex system and the one impacts the other. This is particularly true for our complexion. As the saying goes: The skin is the mirror of the soul. And yes, if something is wrong on the inside–an organic imbalance, for instance–it will show on the outside: the skin.

Acne itself results in mental stress for many patients. It is often assumed that this only applies to young patients in their teenage years, when they are generally preoccupied with how they look and what others think about their appearance. However, most of the patients I see in my daily practice are adults, and I can truly say that all of them experience emotional discomfort, no matter their age and time in their lives. The problem is that skin problems cause emotional turmoil, which is exactly the kind of stress that factors into acne. And so the downward spiral takes its course.

TCM and its holistic perspective understand human beings as the unity of body and spirit. Emotions play a large role in how diseases progress, and particularly impact skin diseases. However, in general, emotions themselves do not cause a disease or weakness in the body. Emotions are a normal and very natural part of our human existence. Only if emotional stimulation and/or changes are too extreme or too prolonged do they turn into pathogenic factors, namely "endogenous pathogenic factors."[25] Then, when coping is not possible, they can cause injury to the internal organs and pave the way for disease. TCM differentiates the foundational basis of the seven emotions. Each emotion influences a specific *zàng fǔ* organ according to TCM. The seven emotions are anger (related to the Liver), joy (related to the Heart), worry (related to the Spleen), melancholy and grief (related to the Lung), fear and fright (related to the Kidney). The intensity as well as the prolonged duration of intense, uncontrolled emotions–everything exceeding the "normal" range of emotionality–can cause dysfunction of qì, blood, and *zàng fǔ* organs, finally leading to minor or major complaints or afflictions, including skin conditions such as acne. Conversely, prolonged dysfunction of an organ usually leads to excessive emotional upheaval.

I would like to illustrate probably the most common pattern in TCM practice: Liver qì stagnation (*gān qì yù jié* 肝气郁结). The Liver (*gān* 肝), governs the smooth and free flow of qì, and therefore ensures balanced emotions. One emotion that can interfere with this free flow is excessive and prolonged anger, rage, and frustration. This emotional setup may damage the iver and interrupt its function of ensuring free flow and balance. When the Liver no longer controls the free qì dynamic, qì is blocked and stagnates. If Liver qì cannot move freely and stagnates for a longer period, the body produces heat which builds up and eventually turns into fire if there is no intervention. In such a case, skin lesions would appear red. If there is fire involved, pimples rarely look pale, and you will usually find the lesions on the upper part of the body, especially in the face. In the patient's treatment, this indicates that you have to soothe the Liver, move the qì, and, if needed, drain heat to improve the skin. However, fire in turn may even cause blood stagnation because fire tends to consume yīn and/or blood. When blood becomes deficient, it stagnates. There is a quite simple analogy: When a river dries out, nothing remaining in the riverbed can move because there is no more water. Like the riverbed, the blood is parched and no longer supplies the skin with moisture. The skin usually becomes dry and tight. So, if you see a patient with severe acne that looks purple, always remember to also move blood in order to resolve blood stasis. The image of the dry riverbed, and its relation to blood within the body according to TCM, is very easy for patients to understand. I often use this analogy in practice. As TCM professionals, we know that we need to tackle the root cause.

Another emotional process might be a cause of acne: Extreme worry, overthinking, and overexertion slow down the transformative and transportive function of the Spleen (*pí* 脾), resulting in dampness and phlegm that block the skin. In combination, Liver qì stagnation, fire, excess fluids, and phlegm also obstruct the channels and collaterals, and often result in accumulations such as nodules, lumps, cysts, and, of course, pimples. These cases will usually present with lesions that are red in color, deep, filled with pus, and very painful. The treatment strategy in this case would be to move qì, eliminate dampness and resolve phlegm, and clear heat and drain fire. The appearance of the pimples changes when blood stasis is also involved. When phlegm and stagnant blood are bound together, they clump and "block the sink." The acne would then appear dark red, tending towards purplish, with larger, nodular lesions that are more persistent in nature. The treatment approach in this case would be to eliminate phlegm and expel dampness, promote blood circulation, and resolve nodules.

In practice, acne often worsens in patients who go through an episode of severe stress, persistent conflict, or periods of recurrent angry outbursts. Skin lesions develop very quickly, and it is really not uncommon for a patient who looked good the previous week to enter the practice with a severe worsening of the appearance of their skin. Thus, practitioners should not wait too long with formula modifications—shorter time intervals are always better in order to provide the best possible treatment to patients with severe skin conditions. Acne is a good example of this.

I would like to share a case from my practice. A young woman in her late twenties came to see me because of mild acne on her face. It was not a serious case of acne; she was still able to cover it up well with make-up. But she was unhappy with her appearance. With every prescription I gave her, her skin got better. However, I also noticed that the young woman did not seem happy and I asked her what was worrying her so much. She told me about her unhealthy relationship, her partner's jealousy, and the many arguments they were having. I listened to her story and then explained to her how the skin and emotions were connected. I did not press her, but advised her to take her time and to think about the entire constellation calmly. About a month later she came back into my practice. She seemed relaxed and looked happy, and her skin also looked very good. She told me that she had ended the relationship, and after this decision her skin improved quickly, and has remained good since then. This goes to show the impact emotions can have!

Asking patients about personal and professional circumstances as well as their emotional state is an essential part of the first and any subsequent consultation. The mental and spiritual constitution is just as important for assessing a person's state of health as TCM syndrome differentiation. Only a combination of TCM and settling any emotional turmoil will make the treatment completely successful. An experienced practitioner, by the way, often does not really have to ask for details because things are so obvious at first sight. The patient's appearance, manner, smell, voice, and, of course, tongue and pulse often give us enough clues. Yet, although we take emotions into account when prescribing, this is crucial: We need to talk to our patients, provide them with an opportunity to reassess personal circumstances, and encourage them to actively take responsibility for their own mental and physical well-being.

Improper Diet

A quick remark on diet (TCM's perspective on food, diet, and acne is detailed in Chapter 8). Times have changed, societies have changed, and so have dietary and lifestyle habits. In general, meat, fast food, and unhealthy sweets are consumed in excess–numerous conversations with patients in my practice show as much. I am convinced that many diseases–including acne–stem from the same negative influences: an unhealthy diet, overeating, and careless eating, pollution, a lifestyle that has an excess of illness-promoting factors,[26] plus a deficiency of health-promoting factors.[27] Affluent diseases are on the rise,[28] and acne is among these. I dare say that, in so-called prosperous societies, living and eating habits unfortunately have little to do with being able to provide the body with the food it needs, but more to do with constant consumption. I very often use the term "measure and middle" in practice to remind patients of a balanced diet and way of life. Less excess in life means leading a healthier one! Eating like a king or queen will definitely promote sickness.

Another major issue is food production and food processing. Modern agriculture and the modern food industry use many chemicals[29] and additives– and the effects are highly debatable and often criticized. Meat production and animal treatment have also been criticized for many years, not only for the lack of animal welfare (if there can be such a thing in meat production) but also for the effects hormones and medication might have on consumers. From my practice, I can report that patients often show reactions to cheap sweeteners and flavor enhancers.[30] One thing can be said for certain: the food industry all too often produces cheap and unhealthy products that do not benefit the consumer.

Therefore, when talking to patients, it is very important to explain how essential a proper diet is. Patients never cease to surprise me when they speak about their eating habits. Thus, I have to explain over and over about how "bad" dietary habits affect the body, and the skin in particular. When the principles of *yǎng shēng* were first developed, thousands of years ago, life and environment was so different from what we know today. Life itself has become faster and demands have changed. We live in a fast-paced world, with an excess of fast, industrially processed food. Everything has to happen quickly, even food intake. Awareness is crucial.

Environment

We are exposed to many things we cannot escape or avoid, be it pollution or chemicals in goods and products we use on a daily basis. For example, chemicals and dyes in our clothes can cause allergies and more serious conditions. However, there are number of environmental factors that can impact the skin negatively and cause skin breakouts such as acne, as listed below.

Weather/Climate Factors

The weather can have a huge impact on the skin, in particular heat and humidity. Anyone who has been to Asia has probably experienced this. Hot and humid weather increases oil production, a known acne trigger. Increased oil production can lead to clogged pores and acne flare-ups. Thus, facial hygiene is all the more important in these climatic conditions.

Dry skin, however, is also a possible factor for acne breakouts. In winter, the skin usually gets very dry due to wind and cold outside, and central heating inside. Dry skin can have microscopic cracks and fissures, in which bacteria can increase and cause acne. Plus, dry skin scales can clog the pores. The skin should be protected diligently in winter, preferably with mild but nourishing skincare products. Mild exfoliation is also recommended to remove dry skin scales.

According to TCM theory, there are six exogenous pathogenic factors[31]– namely, pathogenic wind (fēng 风), cold (hán 寒), summer-heat (shǔ 暑), dampness (shī 湿), dryness (zào 燥), and heat (rè 热) (fire, huǒ 火). Under normal circumstances, if the human body is strong and resilient enough, it has the ability to adapt to climatic conditions and alterations. If the harmonic relationship between human beings and nature is broken, however, the body is unable to adapt to rapidly changing weather or a new location with different climatic conditions. This can be either when bodily resistance is too weak or when there are abnormal or unseasonal weather patterns–which is one major consequence of climate change–as these exceed the body's ability to adapt. In both cases, the consequence is that the six natural climatic factors become pathogenic factors and cause an outbreak of disease.

In acne, the invasion of pathogenic wind is mainly a combination of wind and heat (wind-heat, fēng rè). The mechanism works like this: When pathogenic wind attacks, the upper part of the body (chest and above) is affected first, mainly the Lungs. When wind invades the body–for instance, when the body's defensive capabilities are weakened (weak protective qì, wèi qì 卫气) or after doing exercise–the wind causes a mismatch in the opening and the closing of the pores on the entire body. Sweating, for example, creates a perfect portal of entry for external factors like wind. Pores open and wind can easily invade the body. If the sweat pores are obstructed by cold, yáng qì will stagnate internally. Over time, heat will be produced. Heat accumulates in the Lung channel, and if combined with exogenous pathogenic wind, wind-heat may ascend to the face and subsequently result in acne.

Pollution

One of the skin's main functions is to protect us from harmful substances. Air pollution is a mixture of chemicals and gases emitted into the atmosphere from natural and man-made sources; the latter are increasingly problematic on many levels, of course. This means stress for the skin. Studies provide evidence that acne symptoms might be exacerbated in regions of high ambient air pollution.[32] A disrupted skin barrier can no longer protect from the bacteria that can cause acne.[33] This is why it is essential to cleanse the face before going to bed for a good complexion. A thorough facial routine in the morning and evening is worth a lot.

Make-Up

As much as people want to cover their blemishes, this is usually counter-productive. In particular, the use of oily cosmetics is a major factor that can contribute to acne. These products clog the pores[34] and create a favorable environment for the growth of bacteria. Interestingly, make-up is not the sole issue here; how make-up is removed and which products are used are crucial, too. People might either not wash their faces thoroughly or use make-up removers that are way too oily. Make-up, oil, and dirt easily clog pores, trap acne-causing bacteria, and trigger breakouts of acne. Therefore, gentle but thorough facial hygiene is strongly recommended. Patients need to be reminded that they should never go to sleep without cleansing their face and neck, particularly when using make-up or concealer.

Sun

Prolonged sun exposure increases the shedding of dead cells on the skin's surface. These dead skin cells can clog the pores and eventually become pimples. Heavy and greasy sunblock/sunscreen can also be a negative factor as it leaves a film on the skin. And, of course, sweat production increases in warm and hot weather, creating an environment in which bacteria can multiply. Thus, patients should be advised to avoid prolonged sun exposure, and use little but effective sunblock/sunscreen in order to protect their skin and minimize breakouts of acne.

Lack of Work–Life Balance

Without a doubt, we live in fast-paced times. As a consequence, many people have lost the right balance between work and rest. We often feel that everything has to happen immediately. Too much stress and too little sleep go hand in hand with stressful urban lifestyles. A hectic lifestyle, prolonged overwork, physical strain, or excessive mental labour all set the stage for acne breakouts. Unfortunately, many things seem to be more important than the well-being of one's own body, and alarm signals are all too often ignored. Rest and pause seem difficult to find, although they are extremely important in order to keep our inner balance. Patients need to know that there is a very deep connection between lifestyle, work–life balance, and emotions, and that it is not only their responsibility but also their right to take care of themselves. And it is our job as TCM and healthcare professionals to remind patients of this.

Endnotes

1   In colloquial speech, acne is called *cuó chuāng* 痤疮.

2   The list makes no claim to be complete, but does provide an overview of classical TCM texts.

3   The dates in brackets refer to the periods of Chinese dynasties.

4   Ancient medical books also mention the name *cuó fèi* 痤痱, which means "pulmonary acne" or "Lung acne."

5   The interstitial space is the space (areas) existing between the body organs, tissues, and cells.

6   For example, the literal translation of *jiǔ cì* 酒刺 is wine acne. It is called wine acne when acne is caused by alcohol.

7   This happens after drinking alcohol. It is interesting how often alcohol is mentioned in ancient texts. Acne and drinking have a very close relationship. Keep this in mind for the section on Etiology in Chapter 4.

8   Cold water produces blood stagnation (blood coagulation). Thus, washing the face with cold water, especially after alcohol consumption, should be avoided.

9   This refers to non-malignant tumors.

10 李学川的 《针灸逢源》 中比较有新意的地方在于:他认为 "粉刺" 与 "瘤" 是同类，仅是轻重深浅的不同。

11 This summary does not claim to be complete but should provide a good idea of how treatment has changed throughout time–and in which ways it has remained the same.

12 The formulas are documented without dosages because not all of the herbs were noted with amounts in grams. Plus, measuring units differ in each dynasty.

13 *Chuāng* 疮: sore, wound, skin ulcer.

14 This formula helps the lesions fade away due to reducing inflammation.

15 *Mù lán pí* 木兰皮: the skin (bark) of magnolia tree. Do not confuse this herb with *hòu pò* (Magnoliae Officinalis, Cortex) (same family, Magnoliaceae, but different plant).

16 A species in the genus *Asarum* (family Aristolochiaceae).

17 In ancient Chinese works, there are many recorded combinations that have since been prohibited. For instance, *shuī yín* (mercury) is a prohibited substance and no longer used.

18 Clears heat, resolves toxicity, reduces abscesses, disperses clumps, and generates flesh (heals wounds). Source: Bensky, D., Clavey, S., and Stöger, E. (2004) *Materia Medica*, 3rd edition. Seattle, WA: Eastland Press, p.215.

19 Also known as "Loquat Decoction to Clear the Lung" or "Decoction of Folium Eriobotrya for Removing Heat from the Lung."

20 Interestingly, there is a similar model in conventional medicine called Head's zones, named after the British neurologist who discovered them, Sir Henry Head (1861–1940). In diseases of certain internal organs, regions of altered sensation appear on the skin at relevant spinal cord segments–the Head's zones. These zones can be used diagnostically and therapeutically to influence the affected organs.

21 Unschuld, P.U. and Tessenow, H. (2011) *Huang Di Nei Jing Su Wen: An Annotated Translation of Huang Di's Inner Classic–Basic Questions*, 2 volumes. Berkeley, CA: University of California Press.

22 This is traditional Chinese. Simplified Chinese: 颜 = face, facial appearance.

23 Simplified Chinese: 额头 = forehead.

24 By Sabine Schmitz, 2020.

25 Other internal factors, which in turn induce disharmony between qi and blood and *zàng fǔ* malfunction, are: an improper diet, genetic dispositions, too little sleep, overstrain.

26 Tobacco and alcohol abuse, lack of sleep, work overload, and physical inactivity, to name just a few.

27 Healthy diet, sufficient sleep, maintaining a good work–life balance, physical activity, and so forth.

28 Obesity, cancer, diabetes, chronic respiratory diseases, and cardiovascular diseases, such as hypertension, stroke, and coronary heart disease are considered to be the most common examples of such diseases. Source: World Health Organization (WHO) homepage, 1 June 2018.

29 For example, insecticides, fungicides, and pesticides, to name just a few. Many have side effects and can harm our health.

30 For example, E621: Monosodium glutamate (MSG), also known as sodium glutamate. It is commonly added to Chinese food, canned food, instant soups, and processed meats. A lot of patients report adverse reactions to foods containing MSG, including headache, nausea, flushing, bloating, and diarrhoea.

31 According to TCM theory, exogenous pathogenic factors are the six variations in the climate of the seasons. Please do not confuse this with modern ideas of weather or climate and the Chinese ideas of external pathogenic factors.

32 Krutmann, J., Moyal, D., Liu, W., Kandahari, S., *et al.* (2017) "Pollution and acne: Is there a link?" *Clinical, Cosmetic and Investigational Dermatology 10,* 199–204.

33 *Propionibacterium acnes.*

34 This is also called comedogenic.

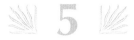

Syndrome Differentiation and Treatment of Acne According to Traditional Chinese Medicine

IT IS ESSENTIAL to note that acne does not present as one single appearance. Acne can present in different ways–with superficial or deep pimples, with or without inflammation. In a narrower sense, acne refers to the pimples that become inflamed. Precise differentiation is very important in order to develop a treatment approach exactly fitting each individual patient. Without this, the treatment will not be effective, as the same therapeutic principle is not suitable for each patient. And this is exactly what many patients are looking for–an individual treatment approach, fitted to their needs. There is no standard treatment for this complex skin condition. This is why before looking at different treatment options, we need to review the differentiation of location and clinical presentation of acne.

Skin conditions are not as superficial as they may seem. All skin conditions are caused by pathogens, and at their root lies an internal imbalance. Precise syndrome differentiation is an essential requirement for effective treatment. In Traditional Chinese Medicine (TCM), the process of syndrome differentiation is called *biàn zhèng* (辨证). All clinical information gained by the four main diagnostic TCM methods–inspection (observation), auscultation (listening), olfaction (smelling), and palpation–are analyzed. More data is gathered through questioning the patient, and details including the location, the clinical presentation, the duration, and the accompanying symptoms such as pain, discharge, and the color of the pimples are evaluated. Since a successful treatment relies on accurate diagnosis, the complex process of making a correct diagnosis according to TCM is essential. Each patient presents with a different origin of the disease and suffers from different accompanying symptoms. Don't forget to have a look at the patient's back and perhaps the chest, as these are also very common locations for acne. It is very important to note the color of the pimples and if they are superficial or deep, at all locations. However, checking the tongue and pulse is another essential part of TCM diagnosis, and this can also provide direction for further questioning, leading us toward symptoms the patient forgot to mention. It is a common experience in clinical practice that patients often add essential information only when reminded of it in some way. Thus, checking the tongue and pulse is very important as a simple indicator for further enquiries and accurate syndrome differentiation.

The treatment of acne employs various treatment strategies and combines both internal and external treatments corresponding with the individual clinical manifestation on the skin. The most common Chinese medicine syndromes that present in my practice and the formulas that have proven to be most effective are explained in detail below, and are listed according to their frequency of occurrence in my practice. It should be emphasized, however, that the frequency of occurrence can vary for different practitioners, perhaps because of local environmental factors, differing seasons, or dietary habits in different cultures.

Characteristics of the skin, treatment principles according to TCM syndrome, and the ingredients, functions, and effects of the different formulas used in each individual TCM syndrome, as well as the first time it was referenced, are all explained in extensive detail. While this primarily serves to increase understanding for students and beginners, it can also serve as a useful refresher for advanced clinicians. Modifications to herbal formulas, skincare, and lifestyle and dietary advice will complete this section, providing a reference that is easy to read, use, and navigate in your day-to-day practice.

Practical Advice in the Use of Chinese Herbs

In acne, as for most other skin conditions, I have found decoctions of raw herbs to be the most effective form of treatment. Although herbal decoctions do not taste good, patients usually tolerate them once the benefits are explained. It has to be clearly explained that the herbs won't taste good in order to prevent the patient's illusion that a Chinese herbal decoction could resemble in any way a pleasant-tasting "wellness tea." Once prepared for the worst, they will come back to their next appointment and say, "You were so right! That tea was the most horrible taste ever, but you know what, after just one week I got used to it and now I don't find it so bad anymore."

My practical hint for very bitter formulas as well as for taste-sensitive patients is to recommend the addition of honey to the decoction, which makes it taste a little less bitter and more tolerable. Patient satisfaction is very important for compliance with Chinese herbal medicine. It is better to drink a decoction with a little honey in it than drink nothing. You can advise the patient that a lukewarm or warm decoction will taste more tolerable than drinking it cold, especially when a formula contains a lot of very bitter herbs. Additionally, keep in mind that bitter decoctions should never be consumed cold, as the cold and bitter herbs will affect the Stomach and patients may feel uncomfortable after drinking it. One hint for making cold and bitter herbs more tolerable for patients with a weak digestion is to use *páo zhì* 炮制. This traditional preparation process, which changes and enhances the therapeutic effect of medicinal plants, has already been explained in detail in the section "Chinese Herbal Treatment Options in Chinese Medical Dermatology" in Chapter 3. However, dry frying (*chǎo*) can be used to minimize the bitter and cold nature of herbs that easily harm the Spleen and Stomach. This preparation method reduces their cold properties and makes them more tolerable for the digestive system, and any qualified TCM pharmacy will be able to prepare it. In conclusion: Raw herbs are always best; don't deviate from them!

Wind-Heat Stagnating in the Lungs
(*Fēng Rè Fàn Fèi Zhèng* 风热犯肺证)
Characteristics

The most common pattern of acne is wind-heat stagnating in the Lungs. In this pattern, acne occurs soon after the wind-heat invasion. Skin conditions caused by wind-heat are characterized by rapid onset, often after an episode of common cold or flu, and are often quick to resolve. The skin lesions primarily appear on the face, mainly cheeks and forehead, and rarely on the back or chest. The skin is red, feels warm, and the acne usually manifests as bright-red, inflamed papules and pustules, which are painful and can itch. Accompanying symptoms may include constipation, dark-yellow urine, a dry mouth, thirst, restlessness, and flushing of the face. If there has been a recent flu or common cold, then cough, breathlessness, and a feeling of warmth may be present.

The tongue is red with a thin yellow coating. The pulse is rapid and floating, or rapid and slippery, depending on whether there is phlegm in the Lungs.

Treatment Principle

Clear heat in the Lungs and dispel wind (*qīng fèi qū fēng* 清肺祛风).

Representative Formula

Pí Pá Qīng Fèi Yǐn (Eriobotrya Decoction to Clear the Lung, also known as Loquat Decoction to Clear the Lung).[1]

Ingredients

pí pá yè	Eriobotryae Japonicae, Folium	12–15 g
sāng bái pí	Mori, Cortex	9–12 g
huáng bǎi	Phellodendri, Cortex	9–10 g
huáng lián	Coptidis, Rhizoma	3–6 g
rén shēn	Ginseng, Radix	1–3 g
gān cǎo	Glycyrrhizae Uralensis, Radix	3–6 g

First Reference

This formula originally appeared in the *Wài Kē Dà Chéng* (Great Compendium of External Medicine, 1665), written by Qí Kūn. It is a very popular formula to treat wind-heat in the Lungs, and in addition to skin conditions such as acne, it is often used for patients who have cough with yellow sputum and wheezing.

Formula Analysis

The chief herbs in this formula are *pí pá yè* and *sāng bái pí*. Both are used in relatively high dosages. *Pí pá yè* is bitter and slightly cold. It clears and disperses heat in the Lungs, directing the Lung qì downwards. *Sāng bái pí* is sweet in taste, cold, and downward-draining in nature, and also drains heat from the Lungs. *Huáng bǎi* and *huáng lián* are used to reinforce the action of clearing heat in the Lungs. Both herbs are also cold in nature which enhances the heat-clearing and fire-draining effect. *Rén shēn* tonifies qì, particularly Lung qì in this case, and moistens the Lungs. Due to *rén shēn*'s powerful action of generating body fluids, it is a very good herb to alleviate thirst[2] caused by injury of the body fluids from heat. The final herb in this formula is *gān cǎo*. It clears heat and relieves fire toxins, but also moistens the Lungs and moderates the harsh actions of the other herbs within the formula.

For readers who are interested in modern research, clinical trials confirm that the ingredients of *Pí Pá Qīng Fèi Yǐn* possess an anti-inflammatory and anti-bacterial effect,[3] which might be essential for treating acne from a modern point of view.

Modifications

For lesions appearing on the forehead, use *yě jú huā* 9–12 g. For lesions on the cheeks, use *fú píng* 9–12 g. *Fú píng* clears heat and dispels wind, and is frequently used for rashes. If there are pustules filled with copious yellow pus, add *zǎo xiū*[4] 6–9 g. *Zǎo xiū* in a relatively high dosage of 9 g is very effective in draining heat, relieving fire toxicity, and reducing swelling and inflammation of the affected skin lesions. It promotes better healing of the skin and can reduce the pain of lesions, and is strongly recommended for patients who say that their skin-healing function is reduced. For severe pustules causing distending pain, in addition to *zǎo xiū*, another effective herb combination[5] is *pú gōng yīng* 15–20 g, *jīn yín huā* 10–15 g, and *zǐ huā dì dīng* 9–12 g, plus *lián qiáo* 9–12 g. Used together, these herbs act to effectively clear heat, resolve toxicity, cool the blood, and reduce swelling and pain. This combination can be used together with *zǎo xiū* to strengthen the effect. If the lesions are closed and sebum accumulates in the pimples, use *zào jiǎo cì* 6–9 g to discharge sebum or pus from pimples that do not open. Remember to inform the patient in this case that the skin can worsen temporarily, as the aim of using *zào jiǎo cì* is to open the skin pores and dispel what is inside the pimple. For dark-red, purplish, hard, and painful nodules, use herbs that cool and regulate the blood such as *mǔ dān pí*, *chì sháo*, or *dān shēn*. One or two of these in a relatively high dose (10–15 g) are enough.

If the patient is constipated, add *(zhì) dà huáng*[6] 9 g. In this case, *(zhì)* means that the herb has been mixed with rice wine and steamed, then dried in the sun. This preparation method moderates the herb's downward-draining and cooling properties,[7] making it more tolerable for weaker patients. If the action of the prepared herb is too mild and the patient needs a stronger action, use raw *dà huáng*. It is important to inform the patient that *dà huáng* might have a purgative effect, and advise them to start with this on a weekend to see if they tolerate it well. It is also useful to advise the patient not to start with the first dose shortly before leaving the house for work, but to wait at home a while to see how fast the purgative effect occurs. It could be very uncomfortable for the patient to need to use a toilet while sitting on the train on their way to work, for example. However, if *dà huáng* is still not enough to move the bowels, add *lú huì* (Aloe) 0.5–1.5 g, which also has a strong purgative effect.

Suggestions for External Treatment[8]

There are many options for external applications. To make it easy and practical for you, I have selected those in which all herbal ingredients are generally readily available. I think it makes little sense to list formulas in which the key herbs are not available in many countries due to species protection regulations or other reasons.

- *Diān Dǎo Sǎn* (Upside Down Powder)[9]

- *Cuó Chuāng Xǐ Jì* (Acne (Wash) Lotion)

- *Jīn Huáng Sǎn* (Golden Yellow Powder)

- *Sān Huáng Xǐ Jì* (Three Yellow Cleanser Formula)

Herbal Washes or Wet Compresses

Please note that the following (and all) suggestions for external use should serve as examples, which can be adjusted according to your own preferences–and, of course, to the patient's individual needs. Herbs can be replaced as required and dosages adjusted. Be flexible!

Frequently used herbs for herbal washes or wet compresses for the pattern of wind-heat stagnating in the Lungs are:[10] *jīn yín huā, pú gōng yīng, lián qiáo, yě jú huā,* or *bò hé.* It is also helpful to inform patients that there are many different possibilities for external applications and a great variety of combinations. Tell patients that their wash can be adapted very flexibly if needed. One very simple example of a frequently used and effective combination in this pattern:

jīn yín huā	Lonicerae Japonicae, Flos	10–15 g
pú gōng yīng	Taraxaci, Herba	15 g
lián qiáo	Forsythiae, Fructus	9–12 g
+/– *yě jú huā*	Chrysanthemi Indici, Flos	9–12 g

This combination is suitable for 350–500 ml of water depending on how concentrated you want the wash to be. If you want it to be stronger, use less water; if you want it to be milder, use more water.

Individually tailored herbal washes with herbs that clear heat and relieve toxicity are best for this pattern. Applied topically, they can help with itching, heat, inflammation, pustules, swellings, ulcerations, and healing of the skin. All these herbs can be used as a basis for external treatment, depending on what else the individual requires. Dosages can be flexibly changed according to the preferred action within the herbal combination. However, while each herb can be used as a stand-alone herb or in combination, only three or four herbs are needed.

Simple examples of frequently used and effective stand-alone herbs for this pattern:

- *pú gōng yīng* (Taraxaci, Herba) 15–30 g

- *yě jú huā* (Chrysanthemi Indici, Flos) 15 g

- *zhāng nǎo* (Camphora) 10 g

- *liú huáng* (Sulphur) 5 g

The dosages listed above are for a wash prepared with about 150 ml of water. Detailed explanations on how to apply washes to the skin are given in Appendix I.

Yě jú huā is useful here not only for its heat-clearing and toxicity-relieving action, but also for guiding other herbs to the face. *Zhāng nǎo* (camphor) must be used with caution, because it is suitable for external application only. Patients should be informed that it is toxic if taken internally! *Zhāng nǎo* and *liú huáng* should be used very carefully for people with skin allergies, and if an allergic reaction occurs, they must stop using it immediately. Additional information on the internal use of *liú huáng*: Although *liú huáng* is suitable for internal intake, it has a strong action and should be used with caution and only in very low dosages.

Example Pictures of the Tongue

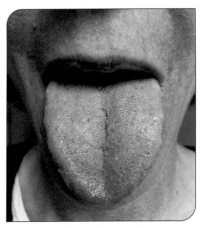

A tongue with a red tip and thin coating.

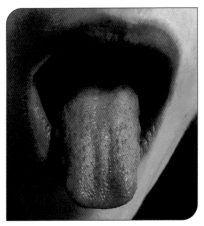

A tongue with a red tip and thin yellow coating.

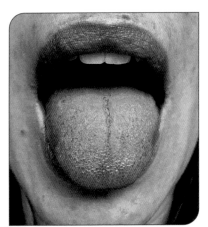

A red tongue with a yellow coating. This patient has had a common cold with cough.

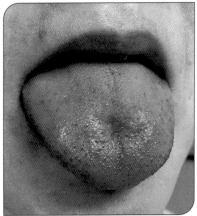

When wind combines with heat, the tip of the tongue is particularly red.

Example Pictures of the Skin

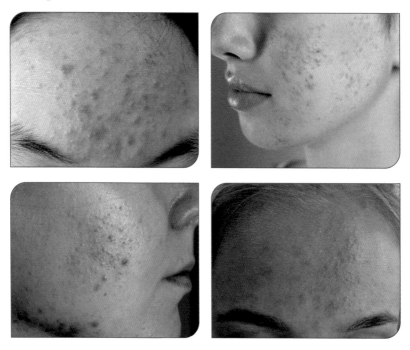

Damp-Heat Stagnating in the Stomach
(*Shī Rè Zǔ Wèi Zhèng* 湿热阻胃证)
Characteristics

Excess oily, greasy, spicy, and sweet food may lead to dampness and heat in the Spleen and Stomach, which can ascend to the face following the pathway of the Stomach channel. It is not uncommon to see this pattern in overweight people who lead an unhealthy lifestyle, often combining excessive alcohol consumption, cigarettes, too little exercise, and unhealthy eating habits. These patients will often love potato chips (crisps) and sweets. Patients may have oily skin, particularly on the face, upper chest, and back. The lesions are usually red, thick, edematous, inflamed, and very painful, with papules, papulopustules, and/or pustules. The pustules are normally bigger than in the wind-heat pattern and the duration of symptoms is longer. The pustules can also vary depending on the predominance of heat or dampness. If there is more heat present, the pustules are redder in color; if there is more dampness, the pustules appear more yellowish. A further typical finding in this type is the so-called "iceberg phenomenon" on the patient's skin surface.

This means that on the surface of the skin only a white or yellow tip can be seen, but under the surface the pimple is very deep and large in size. In this scenario, the skin feels quite painful. Accompanying signs and symptoms may include bad breath, a foul or bitter taste in the mouth, thirst, loss of appetite, constipation, and dark-yellow urine.

The tongue is red with a greasy (sticky), yellow coating and the pulse is slippery and/or rapid.

Treatment Principle

Clear heat, eliminate dampness, remove toxin (*qīng rè, qū shī, xiāo dú* 清热, 祛湿, 消毒).

Representative Formula

Yīn Chén Hāo Tāng (Artemisiae Scopariae Decoction, also known as Capillaris Combination), frequently combined with *Wǔ Wèi Xiāo Dú Yǐn* (Five Ingredient Decoction to Eliminate Toxins) in order to boost the heat and toxin removing effect.

Ingredients
Yīn Chén Hāo Tāng (Artemisiae Scopariae Decoction)

yīn chén hāo	Artemisiae Scopariae, Herba	15 g
zhī zǐ	Gardeniae, Fructus	9–12 g
dà huáng	Rhei, Radix et Rhizoma	6–9 g

Wǔ Wèi Xiāo Dú Yǐn (Five Ingredient Decoction to Eliminate Toxins)

jīn yín huā	Lonicerae Japonicae, Flos	12–15 g
pú gōng yīng	Taraxaci, Herba	9–15 g
yě jú huā	Chrysanthemi Indici, Flos	9–15 g
zǐ huā dì dīng	Violae, Herba	9–15 g
tiān kuí zǐ[11]	Semiaquilegiae, Radix	9–15 g

First Reference

First reference of *Yīn Chén Hāo Tāng*: *Shāng Hán Zá Bìng Lùn* (Treatise on Cold Damage Diseases and Miscellaneous Diseases, c. 219 AD), written by Zhāng Zhòng-Jǐng.

First reference of *Wǔ Wèi Xiāo Dú Yǐn*: *Yī Zōng Jīn Jiàn* (The Golden Mirror of Ancestral Medicine, c. 1736–1743), written by Wú Qiān *et al.*

Formula Analysis
Yīn Chén Hāo Tāng

In this prescription, *yīn chén hāo* is used as the chief herb in a relatively large dose of 15 g. The larger the dosage, the more effective it will be. *Yīn chén hāo* is a bitter, pungent, and slightly cold herb with a fragrant aroma, which clears heat, removes toxins, and eliminates dampness. It is frequently used in the treatment of damp rashes and sores, and many other skin diseases. *Zhī zǐ* acts as the deputy herb. It is bitter and cold with a downward direction of action, and it can effectively clear heat, drain fire, relieve toxicity, and cool the blood. It assists *yīn chén hāo* by guiding damp-heat out through the urine. *Dà huáng*, as the assistant, purges heat, expels stasis, directs downward, and removes damp-heat through the stool. This formula is very small but very effective in the treatment of damp-heat. It is an essential formula to treat jaundice due to damp-heat. However, in order to treat acne due to damp-heat in the Stomach, this formula is not enough to clear heat-toxins on its own, and therefore it is frequently combined with *Wǔ Wèi Xiāo Dú Yǐn*.

Wǔ Wèi Xiāo Dú Yǐn

This is a fundamental formula for treating all types of deep-rooted and hard boils[12] due to toxic heat. It is frequently used in acne as well as in numerous other skin conditions. Whenever skin lesions are marked by swelling, erythema, inflammation, and pain due to internal heat and toxin, *Wǔ Wèi Xiāo Dú Yǐn* is the formula of choice, effectively combining a number of cooling and toxicity-resolving herbs. In this prescription *jīn yín huā*, used in a relatively large dosage, is the chief herb. It effectively clears heat and relieves toxicity. *Pú gōng yīng, yě jú huā, zǐ huā dì dīng*, and *tiān kuí zǐ* clear heat and relieve toxicity. Acting as deputy and assistant herbs, they aid *jīn yín huā* in clearing heat and relieving toxicity, which enables the formula to clear toxic heat from deep-rooted boils. Caution: All herbs in this prescription are bitter in flavor and cold in nature. If taken at too large a dose, or for too long, the Spleen and Stomach may be harmed. Therefore, this formula should be taken only when a strong heat-clearing and toxicity-relieving effect is wanted. When it is no longer needed, stop this formula.

Modifications

To increase the inflammation-reducing effects, add *bái huā shé shé cǎo* 9–12 g. *Bái huā shé shé cǎo* is often used when thick, red, and painful pustules filled with yellowish pus are predominant. If the patient has oily skin, add *shān zhā* and *zé xiè*, both at a relatively large dosage of 15–30 g. *Shān zhā* is also very good for treating abdominal distension. The tongue coating in this case must be thick and greasy–otherwise, don't use this herb. Please note that large doses of *shān zhā* are contraindicated during pregnancy.[13] In fact, many of the invigorating or downward-draining herbs are contraindicated during pregnancy. You may need to inform any pregnant patients that you are using a milder approach, as the priority in pregnancy is to stabilize, nourish, and hold. The harsh approach with many draining herbs that is often needed to treat severe and complex skin diseases is not suitable in pregnancy, and many patients will choose to pause treatment for their skin, then resume again after delivery. For blood stasis, add *dān shēn* at a dose of 12–15 g. *Dān shēn* is an effective herb for cooling and regulating the blood, and is often used for dark-red, purplish, hard, and painful nodules. *Mǔ dān pí* or *chì sháo* are also be suitable herbs to use. Always keep in mind that TCM offers a variety of herbs in each category. If the patient has a dry stool and/or defecation feels incomplete, add *(zhì) dà huáng* 9 g. *Lú huì* can be used as alternative for constipation. If the urine is dark yellow, add *dàn zhú yè* 3 g and *chē qián cǎo* 15 g. If *chē qián cǎo* is not available, *chē qián zǐ* can be used instead with the same dosage. *Chē qián cǎo* (whole plant of Herba Plantaginis) is sweet in taste and cold in nature. It is better at clearing heat and it also detoxifies. The seeds of the plant *chē qián zǐ* are less cold and can expel damp-heat out of the body through the urine. To reduce the cold nature of the herb, it can be used dry-fried (*chǎo*).

Many of the herbs mentioned above are cold in nature and therefore have a tendency to harm the Spleen. In order to protect the Spleen's function, one can use *fú líng* 10–12 g and *yì yǐ rén* 15 g. Both herbs ensure that no dampness remains in the Spleen, which, in turn, protects it. In this case, *bái zhú* would not be effective because it tonifies Spleen qì but has a weaker ability to dry dampness. The same applies for *dǎng shēn*, which tonifies the Spleen but has a negligible effect on draining dampness. To improve the taste of this formula for taste-sensitive patients, add *dà zǎo* 9–10 g, which will also help protect the Spleen. Please don't use *gān cǎo* as it is too sweet and sticky and therefore tends to produce dampness.

If there is more heat than dampness, use *Lóng Dǎn Xiè Gān Tāng* (Gentian Decoction to Drain the Liver) instead of *Yīn Chén Hāo Tāng* (Artemisiae Scopariae Decoction). *Lóng dǎn cǎo* is the main herb within this formula, used in a relatively large dose of 6–9 g. *Lóng Dǎn Xiè Gān Tāng* has a stronger heat-clearing action than *Yīn Chén Hāo Tāng*, so switching to this formula is a very good alternative in cases of severe heat and toxin. In this case, the tongue is red, especially at the lateral borders, which correspond to the Liver in Chinese medicine. The tongue coating is thin and yellow. Acne will present as pustules filled with pus and/or red nodules, typically found at the temples.

The ingredients of *Lóng Dǎn Xiè Gān Tāng* are:

lóng dǎn cǎo	Gentianiae, Radix	6–9 g
huáng qín	Scutellariae, Radix	9–12 g
zhī zǐ	Gardeniae, Fructus	9–12 g
chái hú	Bupleuri, Radix	9 g
mù tōng	Akebiae, Caulis	9 g
chē qián zǐ	Plantaginis, Semen	9 g
zé xiè	Alismatis, Rhizoma	12 g
shēng dì huáng	Rehmanniae Glutinosae, Radix	9–12 g
dāng guī	Angelicae Sinensis, Radix	6–9 g
gān cǎo	Glycyrrhizae Uralensis, Radix	6 g

Suggestions for External Treatment[14]

- *Diān Dǎo Sǎn* (Upside Down Powder)

- *Cuó Chuāng Xǐ Jì* (Acne (Wash) Lotion)

- *Jīn Huáng Sǎn* (Golden Yellow Powder)

- *Sān Huáng Xǐ Jì* (Three Yellow Cleanser Formula)

- *Huáng Qín Gāo* (Scutellariae Baicalensis Paste)

- *Pí Shī Yī Gāo* (Pus Absorbing Ointment)

- *Zào Shī Xǐ Gāo* (Damp-Heat Eliminating Ointment)

Herbal Washes or Wet Compresses

Frequently used herbs for herbal washes or wet compresses for this TCM pattern are: *huáng băi, huáng qín, huáng lián, tŭ fú líng, liú huáng, shí gāo, míng fán, bīng piàn, pú gōng yīng*, and *zhāng năo*. Herbs that strongly clear heat, drain fire, resolve toxicity, and reduce swelling and pain are most suitable.

Examples for individually tailored herbal washes or wet compresses:

huáng băi	Phellodendri, Cortex	10-15 g
huáng qín	Scutellariae, Radix	10-15 g
huáng lián	Coptidis, Rhizoma	10 g

This combination is prepared with 300 ml of water. *Tŭ fú líng* 15–30 g can be added to enhance the heat-clearing process and reduce redness and swelling.

liú huáng	Sulphur	6 g
shí gāo	Gypsum Fibrosum	15-30 g
míng fán	Alumen	3-6 g
bīng piàn	Borneolum	3 g
+/− *zhè bèi mŭ*	Fritillariae Thunbergii, Bulbus	9 g

This combination is prepared with 350 ml of water. The dosages of most herbs are not large, so only a small amount of water is needed. Always keep in mind that the amount of water you use depends not only on how many herbs but also on the dosages you use.

Simple examples of frequently used stand-alone herbs in this pattern:

- *pú gōng yīng* (Taraxaci, Herba) 15–30 g

- *tŭ fú líng* (Smilacis Glabrae, Rhizoma) 15–30 g

- *zhāng năo* (Camphora) 10 g

- *liú huáng* (Sulphur) 5 g

Example Pictures of the Tongue

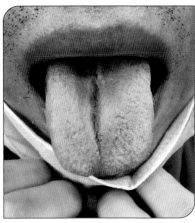

A tongue with a very thick yellow coating.

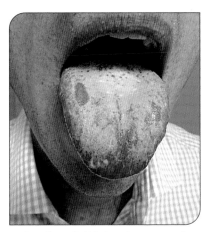

A puffy and slightly red tongue with a thick yellow and greasy coating.

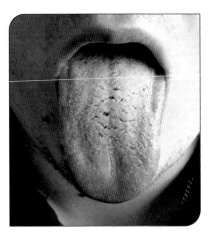

A slightly red tongue with tooth-marks and a thick yellow coating.

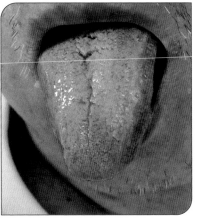

A tongue with a very thick and greasy yellow coating.

Example Pictures of the Skin

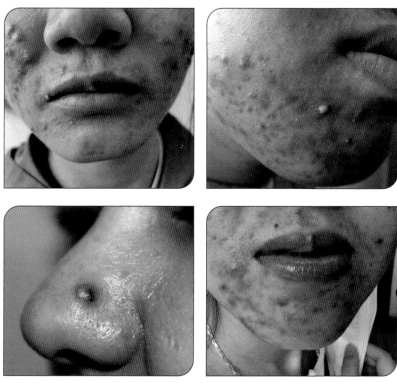

A pustule on oily skin.[14]

Oily skin with thick, red, and inflamed lesions.

Internal Accumulation of Phlegm and Dampness
(*Tán Shī Nèi Zǔ Zhèng* 痰湿内阻证)

Accumulation of phlegm and dampness, if left untreated, can easily develop into accumulation of phlegm and blood stasis (please see the section "Knotting Together of Phlegm and Blood Stasis"). It is therefore important, in this earlier or intermediate stage, to eliminate phlegm and dampness but also move blood to prevent blood stagnation. The transition between these two patterns or stages is fluid, and can be classified according to the color of the lesions. Note that patients usually don't seek treatment at the earlier stages when the pattern is purely accumulation of phlegm and dampness. While we need to be aware of it as a pattern, in practice the picture will always involve some degree of inflammation and blood stasis, and so the illustrations of the skin will be covered in the next section.

Characteristics

If phlegm and dampness is predominant, the skin lesions primarily manifest as nodules and cysts (with or without scarring). The color of the lesions is relatively normal, without obvious inflammation. The surface of the lesions is generally smooth and not necessarily painful. The more blood stagnation is present, the more hard and dark (livid) the lesions become. Accompanying symptoms can include fatigue, poor appetite, loose stools, and abdominal distension. Patients also tend to get a recurrent stuffy nose or blocked sinuses due to phlegm. It is not uncommon for them to have phlegm in the throat in the morning, and to struggle to get out of bed. Everything tends to be very sluggish and slow in the morning.

The tongue is puffy and pale with tooth-marks and a greasy coating, usually white. The more inflamed the lesions, the more likely there is to be a yellowish tongue coating. This applies to blood stagnation too. The more the blood stagnates, the more a livid (purple or dark) discoloration of the tongue and/or purplish veins underneath the tongue can be seen. The pulse is soft[16] and slippery.

Treatment Principle

Eliminate dampness and resolve phlegm, activate blood circulation, and resolve nodules (*qū shī huà tán, huó xuè xiāo zhēng* 祛湿化痰, 活血消癥).

Representative Formula

Èr Chén Tāng (Decoction of Two Old (Cured) Drugs, also known as Citrus and Pinellia Combination), combined with *Táo Hóng Sì Wù Tāng* (Four Substance Decoction with Safflower and Peach Kernel).

Ingredients
Èr Chén Tāng (Decoction of Two Old (Cured) Drugs)

bàn xià	Pinelliae, Rhizoma	12–15 g
chén pí	Citri Reticulatae, Pericarpium	9–12 g
fú líng	Poriae Cocos, Sclerotium	9–12 g
zhì gān cǎo	Glycyrrhizae Preparata, Radix	3–5 g

Táo Hóng Sì Wù Tāng (Four Substance Decoction with Safflower and Peach Kernel)

shú dì huáng	Rehmanniae Preparata, Radix	9–12 g
bái sháo	Paeonia Albiflora, Radix	9–12 g
dāng guī	Angelicae Sinensis, Radix	9–12 g
chuān xiōng	Chuanxiong, Rhizoma	9 g
táo rén	Persicae, Semen	9 g
hóng huā	Carthami, Flos	6–9 g

First Reference

First reference of *Èr Chén Tāng*: *Tài Píng Huì Mín Hé Jì Jú Fāng* (Formulary of the Pharmacy Service for Benefiting the People in the Taiping Era, 1107–1110), written by the Imperial Medical Bureau.

First reference of *Táo Hóng Sì Wù Tāng*: *Yī Lěi Yuán Róng* (Supreme Commanders of the Medical Ramparts, 1291), written by Wáng Hào-Gǔ.

Formula Analysis
Èr Chén Tāng

While some might prefer to use *Shēn Líng Bái Zhú Sǎn* (Ginseng, Poria, and Atractylodis Macrocephalae Powder), it must be noted that it does not resolve phlegm strongly enough, and therefore *Èr Chén Tāng* with modifications is a better choice in this case. *Èr Chén Tāng* is a primary prescription for treating phlegm and damp. It is useful when the Spleen qì is deficient and loses its transformative and transportive function. Its main functions are drying dampness and resolving phlegm, regulating qì, and harmonizing the middle *jiāo* (*zhōng jiāo* 中焦). But let's analyze it in detail.

In this prescription, *bàn xià*,[17] acrid, warm, bitter, and dry in nature, dries dampness, transforms phlegm, dissipates nodules, and directs rebellious qì downwards. It serves as chief herb in this prescription and is best used for thin phlegm or dampness and to open the qì dynamic. *Chén pí*, acrid, bitter, warm, and aromatic, serves as deputy herb, promoting the flow of qì and drying dampness as well as harmonizing the middle *jiāo* and eliminating phlegm. Please note that the original text mentions *jú hóng* (Citri Reticulatae Rubrum, Exocarpium).[18] Most modern texts usually replace it with *chén pí*. *Fú líng*, sweet and bland in flavor, invigorates the Spleen and removes dampness. If the Spleen's function is strong, there is no source to generate phlegm. *Fú líng* also moderates the cloying nature of *zhì gān cǎo*. Sweet in flavor and warm in nature, *zhì gān cǎo* tonifies Spleen qì and moderates the effects of the other herbs. Combined together, all herbs in this formula tonify the Spleen. When the Spleen qì is strong enough, it is able to perform its transforming and transporting function and eliminate dampness. This formula is commonly prepared with the addition of a small amount of fresh ginger (*shēng jiāng*) and dates (*dà zǎo*).

Táo Hóng Sì Wù Tāng

In combination with *Èr Chén Tāng*, this formula is given to move blood to prevent blood stagnation. It is made up of *Sì Wù Tāng* (Four Substance Decoction), which includes *shú dì huáng, bái sháo, dāng guī,* and *chuān xiōng,* plus *táo rén* and *hóng huā*. *Sì Wù Tāng* itself is a typical simple prescription for treating blood deficiency while regulating the blood circulation. Taking a closer look at the individual herbs, *shú dì huáng* with its sweet flavor and rich character is the essential herb in this formula to nourish the yīn and supplement the blood. *Dāng guī* tonifies the blood and helps *shú dì huáng* enrich the blood, but also promotes the circulation of blood. *Bái sháo* nourishes the blood and astringes the yīn. Combined with *shú dì huáng* and *dāng guī*, the action of nourishing the yīn and blood is greatly enhanced. *Chuān xiōng* promotes blood circulation which clears blood stasis and encourages the production of fresh blood. Some food for thought about *shú dì huáng* in this formula: Depending on the lesions, the condition of the tongue, and the desired effect, either *shēng dì huáng* or *shú dì huáng* can be used. If the lesions are redder and a blood-cooling aspect is needed, *shēng dì huáng* is more suitable. If the lesions look relatively normal without redness, *shú dì huáng* may be used. In general, either *shēng dì huáng* or *shú dì huáng* can be used up to 15 g, but keep the dampness-generating effect of *shú dì huáng* in mind. Adding a small dose of *shā rén* 3–5 g can counteract this effect. It is also possible to use *shēng dì huáng* and *shú dì huáng* in combination. In this case, I suggest using 9 g of each herb.

And now to examine *táo rén* and *hóng huā* in this formula. As previously mentioned, it is very important also to move blood in order to prevent blood stagnation. *Táo rén* and *hóng huā* invigorate the blood and transform blood stasis. *Táo rén* is also capable of moistening the Intestines and unblocking the bowels. Therefore, along with its ability to assist in the generation of new blood, it is often used to treat constipation.

As soon the lesions become dark (livid) and harder, this formula will not be enough. It is then recommended to change to the formula described in the next pattern. Please see the description of "Knotting Together of Phlegm and Blood Stasis" on how to treat this.

Modifications

The two formulas described above are used in combination to treat phlegm and damp presentation of acne, but also to prevent blood stagnation. If phlegm is accompanied with heat, add *yú xīng cǎo* in a relatively large dose of 15–20 g. With obvious signs of inflammation, with or without pus or predominant blood stasis, for instance, change to another formula. This book describes numerous alternatives that may fit.

Suggestions for External Treatment

As long as the color of the lesions is relatively normal without obvious inflammation, an external application is not absolutely necessary. However, appropriate gentle skin hygiene is very important here.

Example Pictures of the Tongue

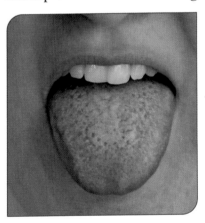 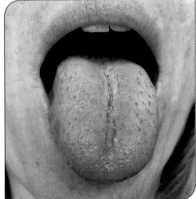

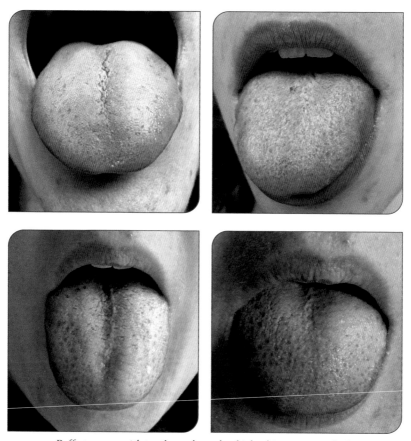

Puffy tongues with tooth-marks and a thick white coating, which
indicates retention of phlegm and dampness within the body.

Knotting Together of Phlegm and Blood Stasis (*Tán Yū Hù Jié Zhèng* 痰瘀互结证)
Characteristics

The onset of this condition is relatively slow and it generally lasts for a long
time. It is definitely not an acute illness. The skin primarily manifests as dark-
red or purple (livid) inflammatory nodules and cysts, and occasionally pustules. The lesions are mainly found on the face, but also on the shoulders and
sometimes on the chest. They are enlarged, thick, deep, and usually hard and
painful to touch. As long there is pus deep inside the inflammatory nodules,
the lesions will be very painful. In most cases, they will leave hyperpigmentation and/or scarring. Accompanying symptoms may be the same as for the

previous syndrome (Internal Accumulation of Phlegm and Dampness), plus irregular menstruation, dark menstrual blood with dark-purple clots, and dysmenorrhea. A note about the clots: The bigger the blood clots, the more severe the blood stasis. The menstrual pain also increases proportionally with severity of blood stasis. The same applies to the color of the lesions. The darker the lesions, the more severe the blood stasis or the longer the condition has been there.

The tongue is thick and puffy, tooth-marked, with a greasy coating, usually whitish. If inflammation is involved, the coating transforms into a yellowish color, but in this case the most suitable treatment may be the formula that corresponds to the next pattern. The color of the tongue is pale and/or purple with dark-bluish veins underneath the tongue. Never forget to check the veins underneath the tongue. If the veins underneath the tongue are purplish, it is a clear sign of blood stasis. The pulse will be slippery and/or uneven (rough).

One more practical hint: In some cases, purplish lips or stasis spots on/underneath the tongue or on the lips can be found. Sometimes, the color is not very strong, so a precise observation in good daylight is essential, in order that these signs are not overlooked.

Treatment Principle
Eliminate phlegm and expel dampness, promote blood circulation to remove blood stasis (*huà tán qū shī, huó xuè qū yū* 化痰祛湿, 活血祛瘀).

Representative Formula
Hǎi Zǎo Yù Hú Tāng (Sargassum Decoction for the Jade Flask).

Ingredients

hǎi zǎo	Sargassum	12–20 g
kūn bù	Eckloniae, Thallus	9 g
hǎi dài	Laminariae, Thallus	9 g
zhè bèi mǔ	Fritillariae Thunbergii, Bulbus	9–12 g
bàn xià[19]	Pinelliae, Rhizoma	9 g
dú huó	Angelicae Pubescentis, Radix	9 g
chuān xiōng	Chuanxiong, Rhizoma	6 g

dāng guī	Angelicae Sinensis, Radix	9 g
qīng pí	Citri Reticulatae Viride, Pericarpium	6 g
chén pí	Citri Reticulatae, Pericarpium	6 g
lián qiáo	Forsythiae, Fructus	9 g
gān cǎo	Glycyrrhizae Uralensis, Radix	3–6 g

First Reference

This formula first appeared in the *Wài Kē Zhèng Zōng* (True Lineage of External Medicine,[20] 1617), written by by Chén Shí-Gōng.

Formula Analysis

Hǎi Zǎo Yù Hú Tāng is a very popular formula. It transforms phlegm and softens hard masses, and is frequently used in skin conditions such as acne but is also very commonly seen in the treatment of goiter and/or thyroid nodules. It is so effective because it not only transforms phlegm but also moves qì and blood. When phlegm and blood stagnate together, these functions are essential, as the transforming action is not enough without also moving. However, let's go into more detail. The chief ingredients of this formula are *hǎi zǎo*, *kūn bù*, and *hǎi dài*, with *hǎi zǎo* being used in the largest dose. All three herbs are salty and cold in nature and have a strong action to reduce phlegm and soften hardness. *Zhè bèi mǔ*, used in this formula as deputy, transforms phlegm-heat, dissipates nodules, and supports the first three herbs in their action. Clinical tip: *Zhè bèi mǔ* is very effective for the treatment of any kind of breast lumps. Don't forget to use this herb in your formula if you are treating a woman with lumps in the breast. Returning to our formula, *bàn xià* and *dú huó* are both warm and bitter-drying in nature for treating phlegm. Both herbs should be used with caution in patients with yīn or blood deficiency due to their drying nature.[21] *Chuān xiōng* and *dāng guī* invigorate the blood and remove blood stasis. *Qīng pí* and *chén pí* relieve constraint due to their qì-moving action. Concerning the heat aspect in this syndrome, even though the acne lesions may show no signs of inflammation, heat is often developing due to the accumulation of phlegm and stagnation of qì and blood, especially if this has existed for a long time. *Lián qiáo* is used in this formula to clear heat caused by constraint. *Gān cǎo* is used as envoy to harmonize the actions of all other herbs in this formula. Together with *lián qiáo*, it can clear heat and resolve toxicity. This condition usually lasts for a long time, and therefore this formula is usually taken for a long time. Instant results cannot be expected, although there are always exceptions.

Modifications

In general, to maximize the blood-moving action, add *sān léng* 3–6 g, *é zhú* 3–6 g, or *dān shēn* 15 g. These herbs are useful when the nodules are dark-purple in color, solid, and painful, indicating more blood stasis. If phlegm is combined with heat, add *yú xīng cǎo* in a relatively large dose of 15–20 g, or *pú gōng yīng* in a dose of at least 15 g. To support the skin-healing effect, add *zǎo xiū* 6–9 g. It drains heat, relieves toxicity, and reduces swelling and inflammation of the affected skin lesions. If the lesions are swollen, filled with pus, and the skin looks redder and is quite painful, add *zào jiǎo cì* 9–12 g and *jīn yín huā* 12 g, +/– *yě jú huā* 9–12 g. For loose stool, add 9–12 g of *bái zhú* or (*chǎo*) *bái zhú*, *shān yào* 12 g, and 12 g of *bái biǎn dòu* or (*chǎo*) *bái biǎn dòu*.

Some patients don't like the taste of algae and kelp at all. I see this quite often in my practice. Here, instead of using *hǎi zǎo*, *kūn bù*, and *hǎi dài*, one may choose another formula. For example:

- Modified *Èr Chén Tāng* (Decoction of Two Old (Cured) Drugs) plus *Táo Hóng Sì Wù Tāng* (Four Substance Decoction with Safflower and Peach Kernel)

- Modified *Shēn Líng Bái Zhú Sǎn* (Ginseng, Poria, and Atractylodis Macrocephalae Powder) plus *Táo Hóng Sì Wù Tāng* (Four Substance Decoction with Safflower and Peach Kernel)

The principle is to strengthen the Spleen, eliminate phlegm, and expel dampness, as well as to remove blood stasis. Don't forget to add some heat-clearing and a few more blood-moving herbs when using these formulas instead of *Hǎi Zǎo Yù Hú Tāng*. Please see above for modifications.

Suggestions for External Treatment[22]

- *Diān Dǎo Sǎn* (Upside Down Powder)

- *Hēi Bù Yào Gāo* (Black Cloth Medicated Paste)[23]

- *Jīn Huáng Sǎn* (Golden Yellow Powder)

- *Sì Huáng Gāo* (Four Yellow Paste)

- *Hóng Huā Gāo* (Safflower Ointment)

- *Huà Dú Săn Gāo* (Toxicity Transforming Powder Paste)

Herbal Washes or Wet Compresses

Frequently used and effective herbs for external washes in this pattern are: *táo rén, hóng huā, dān shēn, zào jiǎo cì, sān qī, pú gōng yīng, gān cǎo, lián qiáo, jīn yín huā, zhāng nǎo, dú huó, dà huáng, xià kū cǎo*. Herbs are chosen according to their ability to promote blood circulation, remove blood stasis, eliminate phlegm and dampness, and soften nodules. A maximum of three to four herbs in combination are enough. Let me give you some simple examples:

sān qī	Notoginseng, Radix	10 g
dà huáng	Rhei, Radix et Rhizoma	10 g
xià kū cǎo	Prunellae Vulgaris, Spica	15 g

sān qī	Notoginseng, Radix	15 g
dú huó	Angelicae Pubescentis, Radix	10 g
zhāng nǎo	Camphora	5 g

These combinations are suitable for 250–300 ml of water.

táo rén	Persicae, Semen	15 g
hóng huā	Carthami, Flos	10 g
sān qī	Notoginseng, Radix	10 g
+/- *lián qiáo*	Forsythiae, Fructus	10 g
+/- *jīn yín huā*	Lonicerae Japonicae, Flos	15 g

dān shēn	Salviae Miltiorhizae, Radix	15 g
gān cǎo	Glycyrrhizae Uralensis, Radix	10 g
dà huáng	Rhei, Radix et Rhizoma	10 g
or *bái huā shé shé cǎo*	Hedyotis Diffusae, Herba	15 g

These combinations are suitable for 300–400 ml of water. If you use three herbs, 300 ml is sufficient. If you use four herbs, 400 ml of water tends to be better. However, it all depends on how concentrated a treatment you want and, of course, how sensitive the patient is to the herbs.

Again, please note that the options of Chinese herbs for external treatment are nearly endless. The redder the lesions are, the more heat-clearing herbs one might choose. The more dark, hard, and painful the lesions become, the greater the proportion of blood-stasis-removing herbs needed, and so on. Other herbs can be added and dosages can always be changed as required. Herbs such as *dà huáng* and *zhāng nǎo* might be possible as stand-alone herbs in this pattern but would certainly not be enough to promote blood circulation and remove blood stasis. Thus, I prefer combinations for getting the most effective result for this pattern.

Example Pictures of the Tongue

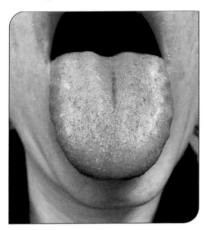

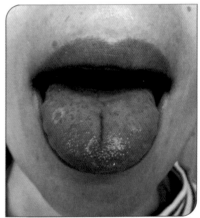

A purplish, puffy, and tooth-marked tongue with a white coating, which indicates blood stasis with dampness.

A purplish, thick, and tooth-marked tongue with a white coating, which indicates stagnant blood and retention of dampness.

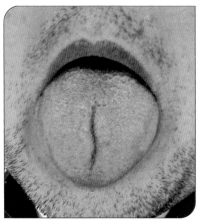

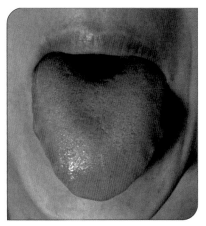

A purplish, puffy, and tooth-marked tongue with a very thick white coating, which indicates blood stasis and phlegm.

A purplish, puffy tongue with tooth-marks and a thick white coating.

Example Pictures of the Skin

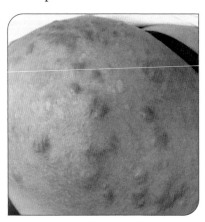

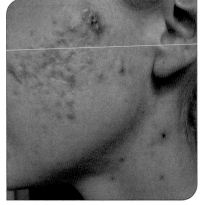

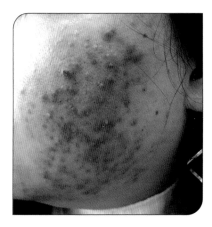
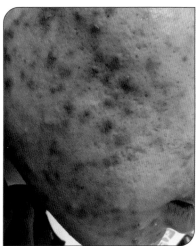

Toxic Heat and Blood Stasis (*Rè Dú Xuè Yū Zhèng* 热毒血瘀证)

Characteristics

When toxic heat mixes with blood stasis, acne appears as deep, painful, and red, dark-red, or (dark-)purple inflammatory cysts, nodules, and/or pustules. This type mainly affects the face, but the chest and the back can also be involved. Both the affected and the surrounding skin areas may be burning and painful due the inflammatory process. Often hyperpigmentation and scarring occur in this pattern as late sequelae. Accompanying symptoms can include a dry mouth and thirst, with a preference for cold drinks, due to internal heat. The patient can have dry stools and dark urination, and is irritable and restless; quite often their sleep is disrupted, as heat is stirring the Heart and the *shén*. This is a particularly severe type of acne where closely monitored check-ups and adjustments in treatment are necessary to observe the patient's progress. At the beginning of treatment, time intervals of one to two weeks are recommended.

The tongue is red or purple with a yellow coating, with or without dark-bluish veins underneath the tongue and/or stasis spots on or underneath the tongue or on the lips. The pulse is rapid and uneven (rough) or rapid and wiry.

Treatment Principle

Clear heat and relieve toxicity, cool and invigorate blood to remove blood stasis (*qīng rè jiě dú, liáng xuè qū yū* 清热解毒, 凉血祛瘀).

Representative Formula

Wǔ Wèi Xiāo Dú Yǐn (Five Ingredient Decoction to Eliminate Toxins) plus *Táo Hóng Sì Wù Tāng* (Four Substance Decoction with Safflower and Peach Kernel).

Ingredients
Wǔ Wèi Xiāo Dú Yǐn (Five Ingredient Decoction to Eliminate Toxins)

jīn yín huā	Lonicerae Japonicae, Flos	12–15 g
pú gōng yīng	Taraxaci, Herba	9–15 g
yě jú huā	Chrysanthemi Indici, Flos	9–15 g
zǐ huā dì dīng	Violae, Herba	9–15 g
tiān kuí zǐ	Semiaquilegiae, Radix	9–15 g

Táo Hóng Sì Wù Tāng (Four Substance Decoction with Safflower and Peach Kernel)

shú dì huáng	Rehmanniae Preparata, Radix	9–12 g
bái sháo	Paeonia Albiflora, Radix	9–12 g
dāng guī	Angelicae Sinensis, Radix	9–12 g
chuān xiōng	Chuanxiong, Rhizoma	9 g
táo rén	Persicae, Semen	9 g
hóng huā	Carthami, Flos	6–9 g

First Reference

First reference of *Wǔ Wèi Xiāo Dú Yǐn*: *Yī Zōng Jīn Jiàn* and *Táo Hóng Sì Wù Tāng*: *Yī Lěi Yuán Róng* see pages 88 and 96.

Formula Analysis

For formula analyses, please see the above descriptions of *Wǔ Wèi Xiāo Dú Yǐn* (Five Ingredient Decoction to Eliminate Toxins) in the section "Damp-Heat Stagnating in the Stomach" and *Táo Hóng Sì Wù Tāng* (Four Substance Decoction with Safflower and Peach Kernel) in the section "Internal Accumulation of Phlegm and Dampness."

Modifications

In many cases, it is recommended to use *hóng huā* in small doses as it has a warm nature. Thus, 3 g of the herb is often enough. However, in cases where heat needs to be cleared, *hóng huā* is not necessarily appropriate. In my clinic, I often use *dān shēn* instead, at a dose of 12–15 g. I find *dān shēn* more suitable because not only does it invigorate the blood and dispel blood stasis, but it also cools the blood. All these actions are needed in this pattern. To enhance the blood-moving action, add *sān léng* 3–6 g and *é zhú* 3–6 g. *Dān shēn* and *é zhú* are a good combination in this case. One can also think about herbs such as *rǔ xiāng* and *mò yào*, at a dose of 3–6 g each. Both herbs have a very strong blood-invigorating action, especially if used together. But please be aware that these herbs are not suitable for patients who have a weak digestion. In this case, please make sure that patients can tolerate the prescription. If not, either decrease the dosage or change your combination. There are many options, so be flexible. For red, deep, and painful pimples mainly on the back, add *tǔ fú líng* 30 g. In order to bring deep, painful, congested lesions to the surface, add *zào jiǎo cì* 9–12 g. For irregular menstruation with brownish blood or old dark blood with blood clots, add *yì mǔ cǎo* 9–12 g.

Suggestions for External Treatment[24]

- *Diān Dǎo Sǎn* (Upside Down Powder)[25]

- *Huà Dú Sǎn Gāo* (Toxicity Transforming Powder Paste)

- *Jīn Huáng Sǎn* (Golden Yellow Powder)

- *Sì Huáng Gāo* (Four Yellow Paste)

- *Jiě Dú Xǐ Gāo* (Detoxifying Lotion)

- *Zǐ Yún Gāo* (Purple Cloud Ointment)[26]

Herbal Washes or Wet Compresses

There are many choices for external treatments as well as simple, individually tailored herbal washes. Herbs that strongly clear heat, resolve toxicity, invigorate the blood, and reduce swelling and pain are the most suitable herbs for this pattern. Frequently used herbs and combinations in practice as a wash or as a wet compress are:

huáng qín	Scutellariae, Radix	15 g
dà huáng	Rhei, Radix et Rhizoma	10–15 g

Boil with about 250 ml of water. As usual, more or less water can be used for the boiling process in order to vary the concentration of the medicinal liquid.

jīn yín huā	Lonicerae Japonicae, Flos	10–15 g
pú gōng yīng	Taraxaci, Herba	30 g
lián qiáo	Forsythiae, Fructus	10 g
yě jú huā	Chrysanthemi Indici, Flos	10 g
+/- *bái huā shé shé cǎo*	Hedyotis Diffusae, Herba	10–15 g

Boil with about 500 ml of water. Herbs can be replaced as required, and dosages can be changed anytime—be flexible.

huáng bǎi	Phellodendri, Cortex	15 g
huáng qín	Scutellariae, Radix	15 g
huáng lián	Coptidis, Rhizoma	15 g
+/- *tǔ fú líng*	Smilacis Glabrae, Rhizoma	30 g

Boil with about 300 ml of water. Use a little more water if *tǔ fú líng* is added.

Simple examples of frequently used and effective stand-alone herbs in this pattern:

- *pú gōng yīng* (Taraxaci, Herba) 30 g
- *tǔ fú líng* (Smilacis Glabrae, Rhizoma) 30 g
- *dà huáng* (Rhei, Radix et Rhizoma) 10–15 g
- *zhāng nǎo* (Camphora) 10–15 g
- *liú huáng* (Sulphur) 5 g

The dosages are meant for a wash with about 150–200 ml of water. Reduce the amount of water if you want to work with a more concentrated liquid.

Example Pictures of the Tongue

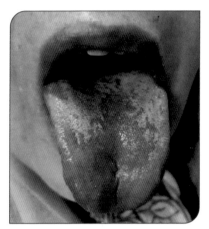

A red and purplish tongue with a yellow coating.

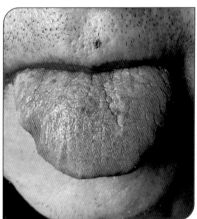

Blood heat turning into stasis and consuming yīn (blood).

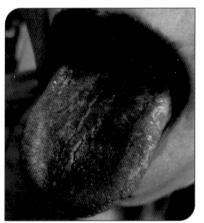

A red tongue with a thin yellowish coating.

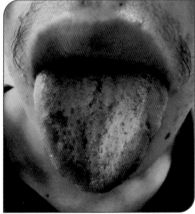

A red and purplish tongue with a thick yellow coating.

Example Pictures of the Skin

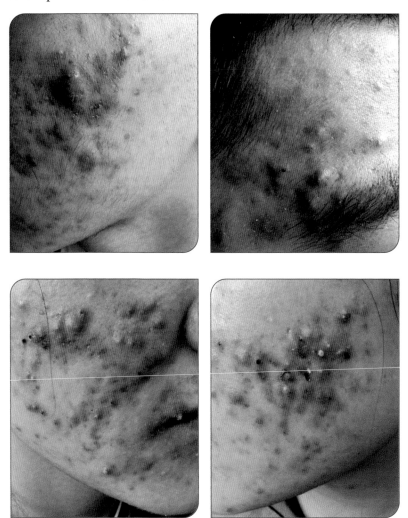

SUB-PATTERNS

In order to provide comprehensive guidelines for treating acne, we need to consider which formula can be used if the above-mentioned patterns occur individually rather than in combination.

Toxic Heat (*Rè Dú Zhèng* 热毒证)

The distinguishing characteristic is that acne tends to appear not only on the face but also on the upper back, shoulders, and chest. The lesions are primarily pustules on a red base that feels warm or hot. Inflamed cysts may also be present. When heat becomes toxic, a greater number of inflamed and pus-filled lesions are always present, along with swelling, erythema, and pain. Scarring often occurs after healing. Accompanying symptoms may be fever, thirst, dry stools, and brownish urine. The tongue is red with a thin yellow dry coating. The pulse is wiry and rapid.

The representative formula for this pattern is *Wǔ Wèi Xiāo Dú Yǐn* (Five Ingredient Decoction to Eliminate Toxins). For ingredients, a detailed formula analysis, and modifications, please see the section "Damp-Heat Stagnating in the Stomach." For constipation, add (*chǎo*) *dà huáng* 9 g. *Bái huā shé shé cǎo* 10–12 g can be added if the lesions are obviously swollen, hot, and painful. This herb is very often used in skin disorders with thick, red lesions. It strongly clears heat and resolves toxicity; it can also reduce abscesses. *Bái huā shé shé cǎo* is very often used in combination with *jīn yín huā* and *lián qiáo* to treat acute, thick, and fresh red skin lesions. For red, deep, and painful pimples mainly on the back and shoulders, add *tǔ fú líng* 30 g. For all other modifications, please see the section "Toxic Heat and Blood Stasis."

Examples of alternative formulas for this pattern, based on the needs of the individual patient, are listed below.

Modified *Cuó Chuāng Jiān Jì* (Acne Decoction)
Ingredients

jīn yín huā	Lonicerae Japonicae, Flos	15–30 g
lián qiáo	Forsythiae, Fructus	9–12 g
huáng qín	Scutellariae, Radix	9–12 g
chuān xiōng	Chuanxiong, Rhizoma	9–12 g
dāng guī	Angelicae Sinensis, Radix	9–12 g

jié gěng	Platycodi, Radix	6-9 g
niú xī	Achyranthis, Radix	9 g
yě jú huā	Chrysanthemi Indici, Flos	9-15 g

First Reference

Zhōng Guó Zhōng Yī Mì Fāng Dà Quán (The Complete Compendium of Secret Chinese TCM Formulas, 1989), written by Hú Xī-Míng.

This formula clears heat and purges fire, relieves toxicity, and cools blood. The actions of many of the individual herbs in this formula have already been described in detail. *Jié gěng* spreads the Lung qì, expels phlegm, expels pus, and raises the Lung qì in order to bring the effects of the other herbs to the upper body. *Niú xī* invigorates the blood and breaks up blood stasis. It directs blood and fire downward. *Yě jú huā* drains fire and resolves toxicity. It is a wonderful herb for treating skin conditions on the face and is often used when pimples on the face are filled with pus. I do recommend using this formula with modifications–depending on individual needs, of course. Please see above for more details about herb actions and modifications.

Modified *Huáng Lián Jiě Dú Tāng* (Coptis Decoction to Resolve Toxicity)
Ingredients

huáng lián	Coptidis, Rhizoma	6-9 g
huáng qín	Scutellariae, Radix	6-9 g
huáng bǎi	Phellodendri, Cortex	6 g
zhī zǐ	Gardeniae, Fructus	9-12 g

First Reference

Wài Tái Mì Yào (Arcane Essentials from the Imperial Library, 752), written by Wáng Tāo.

This is a traditional formula for heat clearing and detoxification, and has long been used in the treatment of inflammatory diseases. Because it clears heat, drains fire, and relieves toxicity from all three burners (*jiāo*), it is a very suitable formula to use when heat needs to be drained from the whole body. In the prescription, *huáng lián* serves as chief herb. It clears fire from the Heart and also drains fire from the middle burner. *Huáng qín* serves as deputy and clears fire from the upper burner. *Huáng bǎi* purges fire from the lower burner, serving as assistant in this formula. *Zhī zǐ* drains heat from all three burners through the urine. The combination of the four herbs effectively drains fire and relieves toxicity. For treating acne on the face, chest, back, or shoulders, the formula must certainly be modified, and herbs that are commonly used for treating red, swollen, and inflamed skin lesions such as *jīn yín huā* and *lián qiáo* should be added. Please see above for detailed descriptions of herb actions and suggestions for modification.

Example Pictures of the Tongue

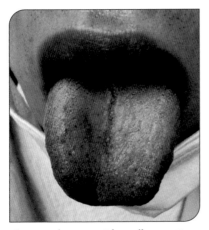
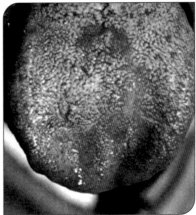

A very red tongue with a yellow coating.

A very red tongue with a thin yellow coating.

Example Pictures of the Skin

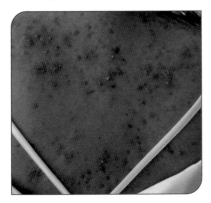
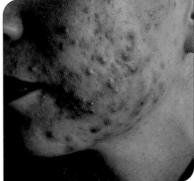

Blood Stasis (*Xuè Yū Zhèng* 血瘀证)

When the pattern is blood stasis, lesions appear as small hard nodules or granular nodules and are dark purple (livid) in color. The skin tends to form scars. Scars and nodules are usually very hard and the surrounding skin surface looks dark purple or dark red. Women with this pattern will usually have irregular and painful menstruation. The menstrual blood will appear dark, with large and dark blood clots. In these cases, the tongue has a livid (purple or dark) discoloration and/or purplish veins underneath the tongue, or stasis spots. The deeper the blood stagnation, the more signs can be observed. The pulse can be wiry or rough.

The representative formula for this pattern is *Táo Hóng Sì Wù Tāng* (Four Substance Decoction with Safflower and Peach Kernel). For ingredients and a detailed formula analysis, please see the section "Internal Accumulation of Phlegm and Dampness." I recommend using this formula with additional herbs that increase the blood-stasis-transforming action such as *sān léng* 3–6 g, *é zhú* 3–6 g, or *dān shēn* 12–15 g. For menstrual pain with dark blood and clots, add *yì mǔ cǎo* 9–12 g and *zé lán* 9–12 g. If blood stasis occurs together with Liver constraint and qì stagnation, add *Xiāo Yáo Sǎn* (Rambling Powder).[27] In this case, the tongue will be pale red or red, especially at the borders, which corresponds to the Liver in Chinese medicine. The pulse is wiry. If qì-level constraint leads to heat, add *Dān Zhī Xiāo Yáo Sǎn* (Moutan and Gardenia Rambling Powder) instead. This formula is *Xiāo Yáo Sǎn* with the addition of *mǔ dān pí* and *zhī zǐ*, an herbal pair that addresses heat (and fire) due to Liver qì stagnation perfectly. Be careful when using herbs with a cold nature. Particularly in cases of long-term use, (*chǎo*) *mǔ dān pí* (dry-fried) and (*chǎo*) *zhī zǐ* is advisable, because the cold property is reduced, but the heat-clearing effect is still ensured. For all other modifications, please see above.

Example Pictures of the Tongue

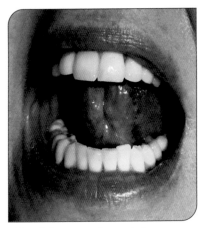

Purplish veins underneath the tongue and purplish lips with stasis spots.

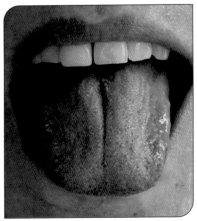

A pale and purplish tongue.

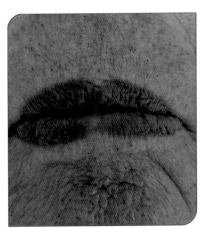

Purplish lips with stasis spots.

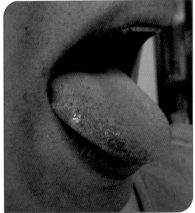

A pale and purplish tongue with obvious stasis spots at the borders of the tongue.

Example Pictures of the Skin

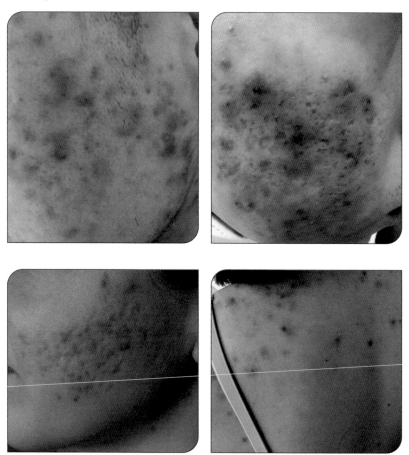

Heat Stagnation in the Liver Meridian
(*Gān Jīng Yù Rè Zhèng* 肝经郁热证)

Another very commonly seen pattern nowadays is Liver qi stagnation with excess heat. Individual living habits and personal environment play an important role in this pattern. Clinical experience shows that stress and emotional factors, such as frustration and anger, are often responsible for the onset or exacerbation of acne. As described earlier, anger will always affect the Liver and its functions. We can observe in the clinic that acne markedly worsens after an upset, anger/rage, or stressful situation. Patients often report precipitating factors such as stress or negative emotions before the onset or exacerbation of their skin condition. Remember that suppressed emotions can harm the body just as much as more obvious and clearly visible emotions. Furthermore, patients often consume alcohol or cigarettes to cope with stressful situations and overwork. Alcohol, cigarettes, and spicy food have been found to be negative factors that can trigger or worsen heat in the Liver and thus exacerbate skin conditions such as acne.

Characteristics

This pattern primarily appears on the face, the cheeks in particular. It may stretch from the outer part of the cheek bone along the ear, to the jawbone, and right up to the neck. As mentioned above, if you see acne lesions on the cheeks, you should definitely pay close attention to whether this patient is chronically angry and frustrated. The acne usually manifests as inflamed papules and pustules. The lesions appear bright red, sometimes accompanied by pain or a burning sensation, but that is not essential for diagnosis of this pattern. Other typical signs of heat stagnation in the Liver channel can be a bitter taste in the mouth and dry throat, irritability, dry stools, or dark-yellow urine. Women may present with menstrual irregularities, dysmenorrhea, or breast distension. Female patients often report that their skin gets worse before or during their period.

The tongue is red (especially on the sides), which indicates internal heat. The tongue coating is yellow. The thickness of the tongue coating will depend on the degree of damp-heat present. The pulse is wiry, rapid, and forceful, which indicates heat excess in the Liver channel.

Treatment Principle

Drain excess heat (fire) from the Liver channel (*qīng xiè gān jīng huǒ rè* 清泄肝经火热) in order to relieve the inflammation of the skin.

Representative Formula

Dān Zhī Xiāo Yáo Sǎn (Moutan and Gardenia Rambling Powder), also known as *Jiā Wèi Xiāo Yáo Sǎn*.

Ingredients

chái hú	Bupleuri, Radix	9 g
dāng guī	Angelicae Sinensis, Radix	9 g
bái sháo	Paeonia Albiflora, Radix	9 g
bái zhú	Atractylodis Macrocephalae, Rhizoma	9 g
fú líng	Poriae Cocos, Sclerotium	9 g
zhì gān cǎo	Glycyrrhizae Preparata, Radix	4.5 g
mǔ dān pí	Moutan, Cortex	9–12 g
zhī zǐ	Gardeniae, Fructus	9–12 g
+/– *bò hé*	Menthae, Herba	3 g
+/– *shēng jiāng*	Zingiberis Recens, Rhizoma	3 g

First Reference

First reference of *Dān Zhī Xiāo Yáo Sǎn: Nèi Kē Zhāi Yào* (Summary of Internal Medicine, 1529), written by Xuē Jǐ.

Formula Analysis

The formula is basically *Xiāo Yáo Sǎn* (Rambling Powder), with the addition of *mǔ dān pí* and *zhī zǐ*. It is a traditional formula to soothe the Liver, relieve qì stagnation, nourish blood, invigorate the Spleen, and clear heat. In this formula, *chái hú* is a guiding herb for the Liver channel; it soothes and regulates the stagnated Liver qì. *Bái sháo* nourishes the blood and astringes the yīn. Combined with *dāng guī*, this action of nourishing the yīn and blood is more effective. *Dāng guī* additionally possesses the ability to regulate blood circulation. *Bái zhú, fú líng,* and *zhì gān cǎo* all strengthen the Spleen and replenish qì in order to generate blood as well as support the Spleen's transportive and transformative function. *Zhì gān cǎo* also harmonizes the formula by mediating the properties of the other herbs. A small amount of *bò hé* soothes stagnant Liver qì and clears heat stagnating in the Liver channel. *Shēng jiāng* soothes stagnant qì due to its pungent flavor and harmonizes the middle *jiāo*. Finally, *mǔ dān pí* and *zhī zǐ* used in combination can resolve qì-level constraint leading to heat as well as heat in the blood.[28] In addition, if both herbs are used together, they are particularly useful if the patient has lesions on the face, as a result of ascending heat, which follows the pathway of the Liver channel. In cases of long-term use, (*chǎo*) *mǔ dān pí* (dry-fried) and (*chǎo*) *zhī zǐ* is advisable, because the cold nature has been reduced, but the heat-clearing effect is still ensured. This makes it more suitable for the digestive system.

Modifications

Dān Zhī Xiāo Yáo Sǎn is good but relatively mild in action compared with the visible clinical signs patients present on their skin. Therefore, it can only rarely be used unmodified, in my opinion. For red, deep, and painful pimples mainly on the back or shoulders, add *tǔ fú líng* 30 g. To bring the formula to the face, add *jú huā* 9 g as a guiding herb. It can clear and calm the Liver as well as subdue rising heat. It also helps that patients love flowers and they make the formula look nicer, a useful effect for all patients, not just those "sensitive" to drinking bitter decoctions. To enhance the heat-clearing effect, one may add *huáng qín* 9 g, with or without *huáng lián* 3 g. Even *lóng dǎn cǎo* in small amounts of not more than 3 g can be used. However, another choice that I frequently make in practice is to combine *Dān Zhī Xiāo Yáo Sǎn* with *Wǔ Wèi Xiāo Dú Yǐn* (Five Ingredient Decoction to Eliminate Toxins). For menstrual pain with dark blood and blood clots, add *yì mǔ cǎo* 9–12 g and *zé lán* 9–12 g. Both herbs regulate menstruation because they invigorate blood and dispel blood stasis. Moreover, *yì mǔ cǎo* goes to the *chōng* and *rèn mài*[29] as well as the Liver channel, and it is not only cool in temperature but also relieves toxicity. For constipation, add *huǒ má rén* 9 g. It moistens the Intestine, nourishes yīn and clears heat. Another alternative for constipation is to add (*chǎo*) *dà huáng* 9 g.

   Dān Zhī Xiāo Yáo Sǎn is one option in the treatment of heat stagnating in the Liver meridian. If a stronger approach is needed, one may use *Lóng Dǎn Xiè Gān Tāng* (Gentian Decoction to Drain the Liver) instead of *Dān Zhī Xiāo Yáo Sǎn*. Clinical experience shows that *Lóng Dǎn Xiè Gān Tāng* alleviates and improves skin lesions because it eliminates fire in the Liver channel, especially in the upper part of the body. The redder and more severe the lesions on the skin, the more emphasis should be put on purging fire with bitter and cold herbs such as *lóng dǎn cǎo*, *huáng qín*, and *zhī zǐ*. By purging excess heat in the Liver meridian, the lesions will disappear. Be careful, as the bitter and cold nature of *lóng dǎn cǎo*, *huáng qín*, and *zhī zǐ* can easily harm the Spleen and Stomach, and these herbs should therefore be used with caution in patients with Spleen deficiency or deficiency-cold syndrome. To minimize their bitter and cold nature, they can be dry-fried (*chǎo*). This reduces their cold properties and makes them more tolerable for the digestive system. The ingredients and detailed explanation of this formula can be found in the section "Damp-Heat Stagnating in the Stomach." For modifications, please see above.

Suggestions for External Treatment

- *Diān Dǎo Sǎn* (Upside Down Powder)

- *Cuó Chuāng Xǐ Jì* (Acne (Wash) Lotion)

- *Sān Huáng Xǐ Jì* (Three Yellow Cleanser Formula)

- *Huáng Qín Gāo* (Scutellariae Baicalensis Paste)

Herbal Washes or Wet Compresses

Herbs are chosen for their action to clear heat, drain fire, ease pain, and calm the skin. Frequently used and effective herbs are *huáng bǎi*, *huáng qín*, *huáng lián*, *tǔ fú líng*, *dà huáng*, *pú gōng yīng*, *zhāng nǎo*, and *liú huáng*. One simple and effective example:

huáng bǎi	Phellodendri, Cortex	10 g
huáng qín	Scutellariae, Radix	10 g
huáng lián	Coptidis, Rhizoma	10 g

Tǔ fú líng 15 g can be added to enhance the heat-clearing process and reduce redness and swelling. This combination should be boiled with 300 ml of water; if adding *tǔ fú líng*, use 350 ml.

Simple examples of frequently used and effective stand-alone herbs in this pattern:

- *pú gōng yīng* (Taraxaci, Herba) 30 g

- *tǔ fú líng* (Smilacis Glabrae, Rhizoma) 30 g

- *zhāng nǎo* (Camphora) 10 g

- *liú huáng* (Sulphur) 5 g

The attentive reader will have noticed that herbs such as *zhāng nǎo* and *liú huáng* can be applied in many different patterns. As long as reduction in pain and swelling, and a cooling and detoxifying effect is needed, these herbs are appropriate. If those actions are not wanted, you may choose other herbs.

Example Pictures of the Tongue

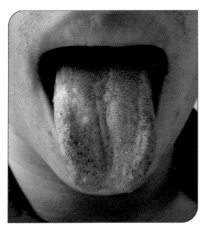

A red tongue, especially at the borders, which correspond to the Liver in Chinese medicine. The tongue coating is thin and yellow.

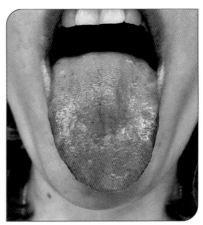

A red tongue with red spots, especially at the borders, and a yellow coating.

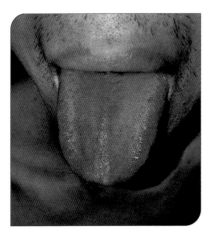

A red tongue, especially at the borders, with a very thin yellowish coating.

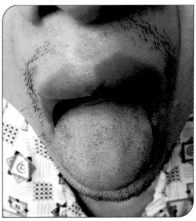

A red tongue, especially at the borders, with a thin and yellow coating.

Example Pictures of the Skin

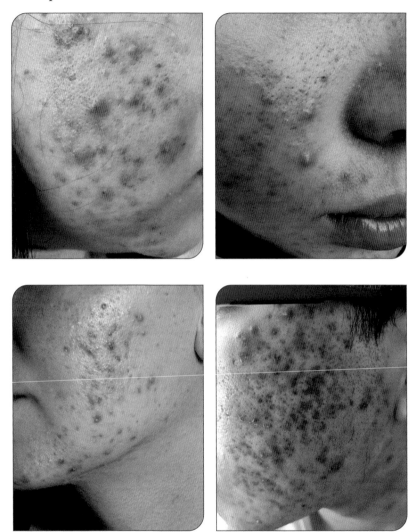

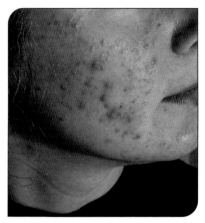
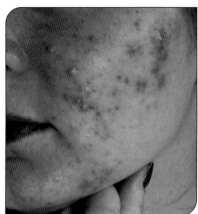

Endnotes

1 While many would think of simply using *Yín Qiào Săn* (Honeysuckle and Forsythia Powder) to clear wind-heat, a stronger and more focused approach to clear wind-heat from the Lungs is needed here.

2 *Rén shēn* is also very useful for thirst in diseases such as diabetes due to extreme injury of yīn.

3 Mansu, S., Coyle, M., Wang, K., May, B. *et al.* (2017) "Herbal medicine *Eriobotrya japonica* formula for acne vulgaris: A systematic review." *Journal of Herbal Medicine 11*, 12–23. doi:10.1016/j.hermed.2017.09.001.

4 Alternative Chinese names: *qī yè yī zhī huā* or *chóng lóu*.

5 Together with *yě jú huā* and *tiān kuí zĭ*, this combination is *Wŭ Wèi Xiāo Dú Yĭn* (Five Ingredient Decoction to Eliminate Toxins), which is a very popular formula that clears heat, resolves toxicity, and eliminates sores and boils.

6 Many books and colleagues prefer to decoct this herb later. I personally cook it together with all other herbs, which is absolutely fine.

7 Bensky, D., Clavey, S., and Stöger, E. (2004) *Materia Medica*, 3rd edition. Seattle, WA: Eastland Press, p.239.

8 The ingredients of all formulas can be found in Appendix I.

9 *Diān Dăo Săn* can be applied as basic external treatment in nearly every TCM pattern.

10 All boiling instructions and detailed explanations can be found in Appendix I.

11 Not available everywhere (e.g. in Germany).

12 Boils: very hard, hot, painful, and deep-rooted sores underneath the skin.

13 Bensky, D., Clavey, S., and Stöger, E. (2004) *Materia Medica*, 3rd edition. Seattle, WA: Eastland Press, p.494.

14 The choice of external applications for this pattern is quite large. Select according to the severity. All ingredients can be found in Appendix I.

15 Source: Shutterstock.

16 This pulse sensation gives the impression of being easily moved, as if your finger is floating on water. This is because the dampness is obstructing the vessels, plus the qi is unable to fill the vessels, giving the pulse its soft quality.

17 Please note that only the prepared herb (root) is for internal use: *zhì bàn xià*.

18 Because *bàn xià* and *jú hóng* can be stored for a long time and have a better effect when aged, the formula was named "*Èr Chén*," which means "two old drugs." Interesting, isn't it?

19 The prepared herb (root): *zhì bàn xià* (Pinelliae Preparatum, Rhizoma).

20 Also called The Orthodox Lineage of External Medicine.

21 Bensky, D., Clavey, S., and Stöger, E. (2004) *Materia Medica*, 3rd edition. Seattle, WA: Eastland Press, pp.324, 413.

22 The choice of external applications for this pattern is quite large. Select according to the severity.

23 May contain herbs that are restricted or forbidden in some countries.

24 There are many effective herbs for clearing heat and relieving toxicity that are available in China and worldwide, such as *xuè jié*, *zǐ cǎo*, or *dì yú*. Unfortunately, these herbs are not available in Germany. Therefore, only those formulas in which most of the herbs are available in most countries will be listed.

25 As basic treatment. All other formulas can be added.

26 May contain herbs that are restricted or forbidden in some countries.

27 *Xiāo Yáo Sǎn* (Rambling Powder): *chái hú* 9 g, *dāng guī* 9 g, *bái sháo* 9 g, *bái zhú* 9 g, *fú líng* 9 g, *zhì gān cǎo* 3–4.5 g, *shēng jiāng* 3–6 g, *bò hé* 3 g.

28 Bensky, D., Clavey, S., and Stöger, E. (2004) *Materia Medica*, 3rd edition. Seattle, WA: Eastland Press, p.96.

29 Penetrating and Conception Vessels.

6

Modern Pharmacological Research

AFTER EXPLORING the effects of formulas and specific herbs according to TCM in detail, let's briefly discuss the pharmacological properties of the most commonly used Chinese herbs in the treatment of acne.

The records of the healing powers of herbs and their mechanisms of action date back more than one thousand years. This knowledge continues to be improved and refined, but has also incorporated modern insight in terms of chemical compositions and pharmacological actions. Each herb has its own biochemical fingerprint, proven by analytical techniques and described in individual monographs. A monograph summarizes a report of the macroscopic descriptions, a list of all the main bioactive constituents of a drug, the pharmacological and biological activities of a single herbal drug, and their therapeutic application. Modern monographs covering an enormous quantity of medical plants enrich the wealth of knowledge about Chinese herbs that ancient doctors gathered thousands of years ago.

Where and when is this information beneficial in practice? Well, this knowledge can be useful for all colleagues who are interested in the latest scientific research about the chemical constituents and quality of Chinese herbs. But it can also be very beneficial when talking to your patients. The concept of TCM is completely different from conventional medicine. TCM differentiates acne into different TCM syndromes, but most of your patients are probably not familiar with TCM terminology, so it can be quite helpful to explain the effect of a single herb as well as a complete prescription in a way that does not require in-depth TCM knowledge. Treatment itself should be regarded as a communicative process, and patients need to be on board with their treatments. If you explain the mechanisms of action in a language they understand, it is very easy for them to follow your treatment suggestions.

Words like "anti-inflammatory" or "anti-bacterial" can sometimes be easier for the patient to understand than "toxins" or "damp-heat." However, it depends on the patient and their interest and educational background in TCM.

A very well-researched TCM formula according to its biochemical actions is *Pí Pá Qīng Fèi Yǐn* (Eriobotrya Decoction to Clear the Lung, also known as Loquat Decoction to Clear the Lung), for instance. This formula contains six herbs commonly used in Chinese medicine for the treatment of acne: *pí pá yè, sāng bái pí, huáng bǎi, huáng lián, rén shēn,* and *gān cǎo.* Studies have shown that the herbs possess an effect of decreasing inflammation, inhibiting *P. acnes,* as well as having anti-androgenic and anti-lipogenic effects. Patients tolerated the intake of *Pí Pá Qīng Fèi Yǐn* well and no side effects were reported.[1] These effects are all essential functions for acne treatment and prevention from a Western medicine point of view, as well as confirmation that the formula is well tolerated by patients. This finding supports the use of TCM as a natural but effective medicine, free from the annoying side effects that can often be seen in conventional medicine.

However, regardless of the results of *Pí Pá Qīng Fèi Yǐn,* there are many other frequently used Chinese herbs that have shown very good results in practice in the treatment of acne. The herbs that I use very often in my practice are listed alphabetically for the sake of simplicity, with their specific characteristics that are important when treating acne—anti-inflammatory and anti-bacterial effects, for example, along with some other interesting pharmacological actions.

Jīn Yín Huā (金银花–Lonicerae Japonicae, Flos)

Main bioactive compounds	Useful therapeutic effects
Phenolic carboxylic acids and esters, iridoid glycosides, flavones, triterpenoid saponins, essential oils[2]	Anti-bacterial and anti-viral,[3] anti-inflammatory,[4] anti-pyretic[5] and detoxicant,[6] anti-exudative[7]

Lián Qiáo (连翘–Forsythiae, Fructus)

Main bioactive compounds	Useful therapeutic effects
Phenolic glycosides, lignans, natural alcohols, triterpenes, flavonol glycosides[8]	Anti-bacterial, anti-inflammatory, supports immunity,[9] anti-viral,[10] analgesic[11] and anti-pyretic effects,[12] anti-oxidant[13]

Pí Pá Yè (枇杷叶–Eriobotryae Japonicae, Folium)

Main bioactive compounds	Useful therapeutic effects
Carbohydrates, terpenes, tannins, flavonoids[14]	Anti-inflammatory,[15] anti-bacterial,[16] anti-oxidant, anti-fungal[17]

Pú Gōng Yīng (蒲公英–Taraxaci, Herba)

Main bioactive compounds	Useful therapeutic effects
Taraxasterol, taraxerol, taraxacerin, taraxacin, vitamins A, B, and D[18]	Anti-bacterial, anti-viral[19]

Sāng Bái Pí (桑白皮–Mori Albae, Folium)

Main bioactive compounds	Useful therapeutic effects
Prenylflavone and flavanone compounds, phenylbenzofurane derivates, other phenolic compounds, alkaloids[20]	Anti-viral, anti-inflammatory, anti-phlogistic,[21] anti-oxidative, anti-bacterial, anti-fungal[22]

Tǔ Fú Líng (土茯苓–Smilacis Glabrae, Rhizoma)

Main bioactive compounds	Useful therapeutic effects
Phenolic compounds, flavonoids[23]	Anti-oxidant, anti-inflammatory[24]

Yě Jú Huā (野菊花–Chrysanthemi Indici, Flos)

Main bioactive compounds	Useful therapeutic effects
Volatiles, flavonoids, glycosides[25]	Anti-inflammatory, analgesic, anti-pyretic[26]

Yú Xīng Cǎo (鱼腥草–Houttuynia Cordata Thunb., Herba)

Main bioactive compounds	Useful therapeutic effects
Essential oil, aporphine alkaloids, pyridine derivates, flavonoids, phenols, fatty acids, sterols, triacylbenzene, lignans[27]	Anti-bacterial, anti-viral, anti-inflammatory[28]

Zăo Xiū (蚤休–Paridis, Rhizoma)

Main bioactive compounds	Useful therapeutic effects
Saponins[29]	Anti-inflammatory, anti-oxidative[30]

Zhī Zĭ (栀子–Gardeniae, Fructus)

Main bioactive compounds	Useful therapeutic effects
Iridoid glycosides, crocins, caffeoyl quinic acids[31]	Anti-inflammatory,[32] anti-phlogistic, anti-oxidant[33]

Zĭ Huā Dì Dīng (紫花地丁–Violae, Herba)

Main bioactive compounds	Useful therapeutic effects
Flavonoids, amides, organic acids, amino acids, alkaloids[34]	Antibiotic, anti-inflammatory, anti-pyretic[35]

Endnotes

1   Mansu, S., Coyle, M., Wang, K., May, B. *et al.* (2017) "Herbal medicine *Eriobotrya japonica* formula for acne vulgaris: A systematic review." *Journal of Herbal Medicine 11*, 12–23. doi:10.1016/j.hermed.2017.09.001.

2   Wagner, H., Bauer, R., Peigen, X., Jianming, C., and Bächer, S. (2007) "Chinese drug monographs and analysis." *Verlag für Ganzheitliche Medizin Dr. E. Wühr, Germany 8*, 51.

3   Huang, K.C. (1993) *The Pharmacology of Chinese Herbs.* Boca Raton, FL: CRC Press, p.292.

4   Yoo, H.J., Kang, H.J., Song, Y.S., Park, E.H., and Lim, C.J. (2008) "Anti-angiogenic, antinociceptive and anti-inflammatory activities of Lonicera japonica extract." *Journal of Pharmacy and Pharmacology 60*, 6, 779–786.

5   A substance that reduces fever.

6   Wagner, H., Bauer, R., Peigen, X., Jianming, C., and Bächer, S. (2007) "Chinese drug monographs and analysis." *Verlag für Ganzheitliche Medizin Dr. E. Wühr, Germany 8*, 51.

7   Nadav Shraiborn, Sirbal Ltd., published June 30, 2015, patent citation US9066974 B1.

8   Wagner, H., Bauer, R., Peigen, X., Jianming, C., and Bächer, S. (2005) "Chinese drug monographs and analysis." *Verlag für Ganzheitliche Medizin Dr. E. Wühr, Germany 6*, 35.

9   Huang, K.C. (1993) *The Pharmacology of Chinese Herbs.* Boca Raton, FL: CRC Press, p.293.

10 Wang, Z., Xia, Q., Liu, X., Liu, W., *et al.* (2018) "Phytochemistry, pharmacology, quality control and future research of *Forsythia suspensa* (Thunb.) Vahl: A review." *Journal of Ethnopharmacology 210*, 318–339.

11 A substance that relives pain.

12 Zhao, L., Yan, X., Shi, J., Ren, F. *et al.* (2015) "Ethanol extract of Forsythia suspensa root induces apoptosis of esophageal carcinoma cells via the mitochondrial

apoptotic pathway." *Molecular Medicine Reports 11*, 2, 871–880.

13 Wagner, H., Bauer, R., Peigen, X., Jianming, C., and Bächer, S. (2005) "Chinese drug monographs and analysis." *Verlag für Ganzheitliche Medizin Dr. E. Wühr, Germany 6*, 35.

14 Rashed, K.N. and Butnariu, M. (2014) "Isolation and antimicrobial and anti-oxidant evaluation of bio-active compounds from *Eriobotrya japonica* stems." *Advanced Pharmaceutical Bulletin 4*, 1, 75–81.

15 Zhang, J., Li, Y., Chen, S.-S., Zhang, L., *et al.* (2015) "Systems pharmacology dissection of the anti-inflammatory mechanism for the medicinal herb Folium Eriobotryae." *International Journal of Molecular Sciences 16*, 2913–2941.

16 Seong, N.-W., Oh, W.-J., Kim, I.-S., Kim, S.-J., *et al.* (2019) "Efficacy and local irritation evaluation of *Eriobotrya japonica* leaf ethanol extract." *Laboratory Animal Research 35*, 4.

17 Rashed, K.N. and Butnariu, M. (2014) "Isolation and antimicrobial and antioxidant evaluation of bio-active compounds from *Eriobotrya japonica* stems." *Advanced Pharmaceutical Bulletin 4*, 1, 75–81.

18 Huang, K.C. (1993) *The Pharmacology of Chinese Herbs*. Boca Raton, FL: CRC Press, p.294.

19 Huang, K.C. (1993) *The Pharmacology of Chinese Herbs*. Boca Raton, FL: CRC Press, p.294.

20 Wagner, H., Bauer, R., Peigen, X., Jianming, C., and Bächer, S. (2007) "Chinese drug monographs and analysis." *Verlag für Ganzheitliche Medizin Dr. E. Wühr, Germany 8*, 47.

21 An agent that reduces inflammation and fever.

22 Wagner, H., Bauer, R., Peigen, X., Jianming, C., and Bächer, S. (2007) "Chinese drug monographs and analysis." *Verlag für Ganzheitliche Medizin Dr. E. Wühr, Germany 8*, 47.

23 Lu, C.L., Zhu, W., Wang, M., Xu, X.J., and Lu, C.J. (2014) "Antioxidant and anti-inflammatory activities of phenolic-enriched extracts of *Smilax glabra*." *Evidence-Based Complementary and Alternative Medicine 2014*, 910438. doi:10.1155/2014/910438.

24 Lu, C.L., Zhu, W., Wang, M., Xu, X.J., and Lu, C.J. (2014) "Antioxidant and anti-inflammatory activities of phenolic-enriched extracts of *Smilax glabra*." *Evidence-Based Complementary and Alternative Medicine 2014*, 910438. doi:10.1155/2014/910438.

25 Wu, L.Y., Gao, H.Z., Wang, X.L., Ye, J.H., Lu, J.L., and Liang, Y.R. (2010) "Analysis of chemical composition of *Chrysanthemum indicum* flowers by GC/MS and HPLC." *Journal of Medicinal Plants Research 4*, 5, 421–426.

26 Wu, L.Y., Gao, H.Z., Wang, X.L., Ye, J.H., Lu, J.L., and Liang, Y.R. (2010) "Analysis of chemical composition of *Chrysanthemum indicum* flowers by GC/MS and HPLC." *Journal of Medicinal Plants Research 4*, 5, 421–426.

27 Wagner, H., Bauer, R., Peigen, X., Jianming, C., and Bächer S. (1997) "Chinese drug monographs and analysis." *Verlag für Ganzheitliche Medizin Dr. E. Wühr, Germany 1*, 6.

28 Wagner, H., Bauer, R., Peigen, X., Jianming, C., and Bächer S. (1997) "Chinese drug monographs and analysis." *Verlag für Ganzheitliche Medizin Dr. E. Wühr, Germany 1*, 6.

29 Wang, G., Liu, Y., Wang, Y., and Gao, W. (2018) "Effect of Rhizoma Paridis saponin on the pain behavior in a mouse model of cancer pain." *RSC Advances (The Royal Society of Chemistry) 31*, 17060–17072.

30 Wang, G., Liu, Y., Wang, Y., and Gao, W. (2018) "Effect of Rhizoma Paridis saponin on the pain behavior in a mouse model of cancer pain." *RSC Advances (The Royal Society of Chemistry) 31*, 17060–17072.

31 Wagner, H., Bauer, R., Peigen, X., Jianming, C., and Bächer, S. (2004) "Chinese drug monographs and analysis." *Verlag für Ganzheitliche Medizin Dr. E. Wühr, Germany 5*, 22.

32 Fu, Y., Liu, B., Liu, J., Liu, Z. *et al.* (2012) "Geniposide, from *Gardenia jasminoides Ellis*, inhibits the inflammatory response in the primary mouse macrophages and mouse models." *International Immunopharmacology 14*, 4, 792–798.

33 Wagner, H., Bauer, R., Peigen, X., Jianming, C., and Bächer S. (2004) Chinese drug monographs and analysis." *Verlag für Ganzheitliche Medizin Dr. E. Wühr, Germany* 5, 22.

34 Bensky, D., Clavey, S., and Stöger, E. (2004) *Materia Medica*, 3rd edition. Seattle, WA: Eastland Press, p.166.

35 Muluye, R.A., Bian, Y., and Alemu, P.N. (2014) "Anti-inflammatory and antimicrobial effects of heat-clearing Chinese herbs: A current review." *Journal of Traditional and Complementary Medicine* 4, 2, 93–98.

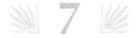

Useful Advice About the Course and Prognosis of Treatment

PATIENCE—A VERY IMPORTANT word to tell your patients! Treating acne takes time and patience. A significant number of patients have consulted a Western dermatologist and taken conventional drugs and topical acne treatments before they come to us for treatment with TCM. Plus, the majority of the patients we see in a TCM practice don't present with mild acne. Most of them have a serious skin condition, lasting for a very long time.

There are certain rules of thumb in the treatment of acne patients.

Acne patients in acute stages or with very serious skin conditions must be treated and monitored continuously without breaks. In the beginning, two or three weeks of taking the herbs daily is recommended. If there is no improvement after that, the prescription needs to be changed, assuming, of course, that the patient has complied with all instructions. If the treatment is followed too nonchalantly, the desired effect will not occur. And if dietary advice is not followed strictly, treatment success will also be difficult. Patients should be disciplined with changes in diet, as it will definitely improve their results. We will come to diet later, in Chapter 8.

- Early stages: Acne is always easier to treat and faster to resolve when it is in the early stages and hasn't yet had a chance to become chronic. The pattern "Wind-Heat Stagnating in the Lung" is a very good example of acne in the early stages. Moreover, shallow red scarring in the early stages of acne will be easier to treat than old, deep, and dark-colored scars.

- Later/chronic stage: If the disease lasts longer, it is always more difficult to treat and, of course, the treatment takes much longer. The patterns of "Damp-Heat Stagnating in the Stomach" as well as "Knotting Together of Phlegm and Blood Stasis" are examples of patterns that are longer-lasting or chronic. The same applies for scarring. The longer scars are present, the harder they are to treat and the longer the treatment will take. It is best to give patients a realistic outlook on treating scars to prevent their disappointment when the scars take a long time to treat and might not resolve completely.

- Nodules: Acne nodules are larger and more serious than a typical pimple and affect deeper layers of the skin. They are hard, very painful, and difficult to resolve. Nodular acne can be tough to treat. Because acne nodules usually last a long time, treatment can take months.

- Superficial papules: An acne papule looks like a red bump on the skin. It feels soft and it is easier to dissolve than a hard and deep nodule. Thus, the treatment takes a shorter period of time. However, acne papules–or pimples, as they are colloquially known–often turn into pustules. Then the treatment will understandably take longer.

Can the Skin Appearance Worsen During Treatment?

Yes, sometimes it can. Patients must be aware of this fact but also that it's not necessarily a bad sign. Sometimes there can be an aggravation before everything gets better. Fortunately, I rarely see that in my practice. However, I would like to give advice on the use of *zào jiǎo cì*. The aim of using *zào jiǎo cì* is to open the skin pores and dispel what is inside the pimple, a necessary step for the pimple to resolve. Thus, it is quite logical that a pimple looks worse for a short time. If patients are not informed about this process, they may be worried and also think that the treatment is not helping and their skin is even getting worse. I have found that if this mechanism is well explained, patients understand and will go along with it. However, that's the way it is with all treatment processes: the better informed that patients are, the less they worry when things appear to get worse.

Treatment Course

It is crucial to inform your patient about the duration of treatment. Again, while acne is one of the most common skin diseases, it can be difficult to treat, even in TCM. Be sincere and explain this to your patient. Trust is an equally important aspect in the therapy. Chronic and stubborn skin diseases have evolved over many years. Thus, instant results cannot be expected, but small changes will occur as treatment progresses. A rule of thumb is one month of treatment for every one year of illness. For chronic and severe types of acne, this is a very realistic rule to give to your patient. Of course, skin can often improve faster, and, yes, I often see more rapid successes, especially in patients with acute acne that has not lasted very long. However, do not offer any illusions because there is much more going on in the patient's life that plays a role in improvement as well as aggravation, such as stress, emotions, environmental factors, etc. You need to confidently represent your position, because this is the truth. We, as TCM doctors, cannot work miracles in weeks and achieve an outcome that conventional medicine has not achieved in several years. Also, compared with the harsh drugs and aggressive topical treatments patients may have already used, a natural medicine like TCM works gently and may take a little longer, but is effective and, above all, sustainable.

- If the skin is smooth, and all pimples and nodules are gone, the patient can stop taking the herbs.

- If there are still skin discolorations, nodules, even small hardenings under the skin, the patient should continue with treatment. It is always a mistake to stop treatment too early. Patients must have patience to avoid relapses. Also, they shouldn't fall back into previous habits that aggravate their skin, especially if they think everything is now good. Unfortunately, people tend to do this. Remind your patients that this will be to their disadvantage!

In conclusion, a good and realistic benchmark you can offer your patients is a minimum of three to four months of treatment with Chinese herbal medicine for chronic and stubborn acne. If the acne is very deep and the nodules are dark purple, it will take at least six months. Scars are always extremely difficult to treat, especially if they have been persisting for a long time. In any case, the treatment should be started as early as possible to avoid scarring. If already existing, one can usually improve but not completely remove them. If your patient trusts you, they will be patient in the course of treatment, and compliance is ensured as well.

8

Preventive Healthcare: Dietary, Lifestyle, and Skincare Advice

Diet

"You are what you eat!" We know that following a healthy diet can definitely help us remain healthy and in good shape. We also know that this can be a challenge. However, just as diet and lifestyle habits can worsen a skin disease, they can also improve the skin's appearance; and acne is a very good example. We know that the effects of a "bad" diet accumulate over time and should be seen in a long-term context. The issue is not just the quality of food but also the quantity; irregular food consumption is also a factor. The following section lists the foods that should be avoided and provides preferable alternatives. In addition, it details information on eating habits and other practical tips we can share with our patients.

Always keep in mind that patients have the ability to speed their skin's healing at home if we make them aware of their own responsibility in their healing process. Or they may contribute to the aggravation of their skin disease if they follow an inappropriate diet and lifestyle habits.

General Guidelines

Certainly, doctors and health experts from different fields have different perspectives on food and thus different dietary recommendations. However, in TCM (and many other nutritional philosophies agree) the general guidelines for patients are:

- Eat only when hungry.

- Stop before feeling completely full.

- Have three meals a day (warm food if possible).

- Do not eat too late in the evening (ideally not after 6 p.m.).

Pungent and Spicy Foods

Pepper, garlic, chili, curry, and other pungent spices tend to produce internal heat, so they should be avoided. Patients with acne often tell me that they love and crave spicy, oily, and greasy foods, often accompanied by alcoholic drinks. Yet this combination is probably the worst possible eating pattern for them. These foods are an ideal breeding ground for dampness, which transforms into heat. The resulting damp-heat in the Stomach (*wèi* 胃) and Intestines cannot be transformed by the Spleen and Stomach, nor can the bowel overcome the stagnation and eliminate the imbalance. The damp-heat has to go somewhere, so it rises to the upper body and mainly manifests as acne on the face, chest, back, and shoulders. For acne, it is particularly important to stop–or at least heavily restrict–consumption of alcohol, cigarettes, and coffee, as well as oily and spicy food. Patients should preferably eat mildly spiced food, and steam their food instead of roasting and frying in excess oil.

In the wind-heat syndrome, foods that help nourish the Lungs according to TCM are recommended, such as pear, peach, carrots, or white mushrooms. Cooling food with a sweet taste will help clear heat and moisten the Lungs– for example, apple, watermelon, bamboo shoots, pumpkin, and some algae. Other heat-clearing food is recommended, such as green tea, mint, radish, or mung beans. When there is damp-heat, patients should avoid spicy and greasy foods. Fresh fruits and vegetables that cool heat in the Spleen and Stomach are preferable instead: apples, pear, honeydew melon, watermelon, lime, mint, cucumber, radish, tomatoes, or soybeans–to mention just a few. Foods that can resolve dampness can also be beneficial, such as cherries or kohlrabi.

Sugar and Sweets

As a society, we consume too much sugar and sweet foods on a daily basis. The same process occurs as described above. A weakened Spleen no longer transforms and transports properly, and dampness develops, followed by phlegm and so on. Sugar, and in particular sweets, are strictly forbidden if a patient has serious acne! This also applies to soft drinks such cola and lemonade.

There was one patient with acne inversa whom I advised to completely avoid sweets and dairy products. He followed my advice and his skin improved significantly. The Western dermatologist had recommended tissue excision to this patient. Thanks to his change in diet and the intake of Chinese herbs, this form of invasive treatment was luckily no longer necessary. Another patient with acne went through the opposite. His skin condition was relatively stable after a few months of treatment with Chinese herbs. One day, he came back to my practice and told me that he had been experiencing a lot of stress and frustration due to his job change. Thus, his diet had not been the best recently. He noticed that when he had eaten potato chips and sweets in the evening, his skin drastically worsened the very next day, which was the reason he returned to my practice. These are just two examples that show that a skin condition can improve by changing dietary habits but can also worsen rapidly after consuming bad food.

Dairy

The consumption of dairy products in the Western world is high.[1] This trend seems to be expanding into the Asian world: I have observed that products from cow's milk, including milk, yogurt, and cheese, are consumed more. Whatever the reason–global trends and advertising, or corporations seeking new markets–from a TCM point of view, this is an unfortunate development.

Chinese medicine considers cow's milk as cooling and damp-forming, especially if consumed in excess. When we look at acne, the nature and consistency of the pimples clearly indicate that anything that produces damp and phlegm should be avoided. It can be helpful when talking to patients with acne to explain how the Spleen works according to Chinese medicine. Dairy products slow down digestive and absorptive functions, resulting in excess fluids and phlegm that block the skin. Thus, cow's milk products should be strictly avoided by those who have serious acne.

However, when it comes to advising patients to avoid milk and dairy products, I frequently hear the sentence "But I like it!"–it is the same with sweets, of course. Show understanding but know that it will likely prove worthwhile to educate the patient and explain the effects of dairy products in their body. The other response to this kind of advice is "I can't do that!" What they actually mean is that they do not want to. We need to accept that change is difficult for many patients but also tell them straight up that they shed their responsibility by claiming change is impossible. Many people are afraid of change, although nature–including our physical body–is in the process of constant change. To make it easier for patients, make suggestions that they can easily adopt without having to change their routines completely. Fortunately, our modern society offers so many alternatives to products that we can usually find a solution for everything. Patients can substitute cow's milk cheese with sheep's or goat's milk cheese. According to TCM theory, both are easier to digest. Tell them about alternative options for milk: almond, rice, soy, or oat milk.

By the way, many adult patients tell me that they still drink a big glass of milk every day, despite the fact that milk is really not meant to be a beverage. Many people still believe that cow's milk contains a lot of calcium and that it is good for them. But if this was the case, why is the rate of osteoporosis in Asian people not significantly higher than in Caucasians? Many people have been told all their lives to drink milk for strong bones, but the truth is that most industrially advanced countries–such as the US, Australia, New Zealand, and most Western European nations–have higher fracture rates, yet consume more dairy products than the rest of the world. Meanwhile, the people in much of Asia and Africa consume little or no milk (after weaning), few dairy products, and next to no calcium supplements, and their fracture rates are 50 to 70% lower.[2] I usually tell patients that calcium as an essential mineral is important for good health, but bone health does not depend on calcium alone. Moreover, I show them a table with natural calcium sources, and patients are usually surprised that cow's milk is not in the top spot. Many foods like vegetables (including kale, broccoli, fennel, spinach), algae, or sardines contain as much if not more calcium than cow's milk products. Debunk this myth for the benefit of your patients.

Fā Wù 发物

From the traditional TCM viewpoint, some foods are classified as *fā wù* 发物. *Fā* means to emit and *wù* means a material or substance. *Fā wù* describes a specific category of food in Chinese medicine that increases or worsens disease rather than prevents it, and *fā wù* food tends to be hot and stimulating. In the case of red-colored skin lesions in acne, heat is already predominant. When *fā wù* food is consumed, it adds even more heat to the pre-existing heat, and thus makes the skin worse. The following table provides an overview of which foods are considered *fā wù* in acne and should be avoided.[3]

Foods to avoid	Pathogenic mechanisms that make acne worse
High-fat foods–e.g. cream, offal, fatty meat, eggs	Produce internal heat, which in turn will aggravate pre-existing internal heat
High-carb foods: • dairy (e.g. milk, yogurt, ice cream) • grains (e.g. bread, crackers) • sugary sweets (e.g. candy, cookies, other desserts) • starchy vegetables (e.g. potatoes)	Cause elevated metabolism in the body, which increases the secretion of sebaceous glands and results in acne
Seafood–e. g. shrimps or crabs	Triggers allergic reactions and aggravates acne by increasing inflammation of the sebaceous glands
Spicy food and stir-fried food	Warm/hot in nature with drying properties, thus always tend to generate heat and fire inside the body, which will aggravate acne
Tonic foods–e. g. lamb, chicken	Heating in nature and thus easily trigger acne

This knowledge might also be helpful in other skin diseases such as psoriasis, eczema, and urticaria.

Bowel Movements and Exercise

The patient should keep in mind that a regular bowel movement is essential–at least once a day. Constipation is an issue that needs to be addressed. If the stool is too dry or irregular, the heat within the body cannot escape, which makes the skin worse. Thus, regular bowel movements help relieve acne by expelling heat from the body. If the patient is constipated, it is recommended to treat the constipation first. Once this has been done successfully, address the other aspects. The patient should understand how important this is, even if they have come to regard constipation as "normal."

In general, the patient should maintain a stable mood, have enough rest and sleep, and avoid overexertion with exercise until the condition improves. The latter is also a myth we need to debunk. Exercise is good for our body, but physical strain is not. Our society (from PE at school to the fitness culture) too often claims that we need to push ourselves to the point of overexertion. Yet patients need to learn to listen to their bodies and know when they need rest, when they need light exercise, and when they are fit enough for more intense training.

Practical Advice on Patient Communication

The right nutrition has such positive effects on the patient's skin that dietary advice is essential. When advising patients, it is very helpful not only to list the individual products that need to be avoided, but also to explain how the Spleen works according to Chinese medicine, and how certain foods slow down its transformative and transportive functions. Give every patient a simple but clear overview of these principles, in a language that they can grasp. In my experience, however, being too strict and dogmatic in our recommendations can be counterproductive. Moreover, complicated technical language and too much information at the beginning can be overwhelming, and sometimes even cause stress–it is your task to know the complex mechanisms at work and be able to convey them in a simple and understandable manner.

Also, let patients know that dietary changes will not show an effect overnight but it will take time. Patients often complain: "I have not eaten this or that for two weeks and I have not seen any changes!" We need to let patients know that dietary changes often take a minimum of four to six weeks to show an effect. If your patients manage to stick to the dietary changes for this period of time, the results are often impressive–the skin appearance improves significantly, with fewer pimples and less inflammation, pain, and skin discoloration.

It is essential that patients understand how food and health are related. This will make it easier to follow your advice. One goal must be to enable patients to enjoy food, rather than simply consume it. Most importantly, an improved diet in combination with an individually tailored Chinese herbal prescription shows very good results in the treatment of skin diseases such as acne.

Skincare

Skincare in Ancient China

Caring for acne-prone skin requires more than just slathering on blemish-covering products. It involves the right skincare routine, along with diet and lifestyle changes. This was already known in ancient China. Beauty has always played a major role in Chinese culture and people have always paid great attention to facial beauty. One of the earliest cosmetic methods recorded in Chinese language was "washing the face." In ancient times, people attached great importance to thorough cleaning and care of the skin. While the TCM doctor mainly treats the patient internally (with Chinese herbal medicine), it is also very important that the patient cares for their skin correctly at home. Many books on TCM dermatology have covered this topic over time. I have summarized some suggestions below from a very important ancient book, the *Pǔ Jì Fāng* (Prescriptions for Universal Relief, also known as The Universal Relieving Prescriptions).[4] This book is the most extensive collection of prescriptions and methods of treatment in TCM in Chinese history, containing over 61,739 prescriptions in 168 volumes. Compiled by Zhū Sù *et al.*, this book was published in 1406 under the leadership of Emperor Zhū Dì, the third emperor of China's Míng Dynasty.[5]

Below are three examples[6] of face washing and facial masks.

Wǔ Bèi Zǐ Gāo (Nutgall Paste) for Facial Acne

> *wǔ bèi zǐ* 30 g, *lòu lú* 30 g, *huáng bǎi* 30 g

For application, grind the ingredients to a fine powder, mix them together with honey, and apply as a facial mask to the skin. Ideally, all affected skin parts should be covered with the mask. Please note that no application times are mentioned; however, I suggest leaving the mask on the skin for about 30 minutes.

Gǎo Běn Sǎn (Ligustici Sinensis Powder) for Facial Acne

> *gǎo běn, qiān niú zǐ, hēi dòu, zào jiǎo cì* (all herbs in equal dosage; quantities depend on the desired consistency)

For application, grind the ingredients to a fine powder, mix them together with honey, and apply as a facial mask to the skin. All affected skin parts should be covered with the mask. Again, no application times are mentioned; I suggest leaving the mask on the skin for about 30 minutes.

Jiāng Cán Sǎn (Silkworm Powder) Acne Wash

> *jiāng cán* 30 g, *bái zhǐ* 30 g, *gǎo běn* 30 g

For application, grind the ingredients to a fine powder, mix with water, and use as a wash. It is not mentioned whether the herbs should be cooked or not. I do recommend soaking the herbs in 500 ml of water for 15–20 minutes. Bring the herbs to a boil and then reduce to a low heat, allowing the herbs to simmer slowly for approximately 15 minutes. Strain the liquid. For application, use the liquid as a wash or a wet compress for at least 15 minutes, once or twice a day on the affected skin lesions.

All of these formulas can still be used today if well explained to the patient. Everything is easy to do at home. That has always been the advantage of TCM: simple, practical, down-to-earth!

Modern Skincare Tips

In the case of clinically acute acne, cosmetic measures are always used in addition to medical therapy. Cleaning and care should be adapted to the skin's individual needs. Skin cleansing and dermatological procedures are primarily aimed at removing dirt and cell residues as well as regulating sebum production, in order to reduce acne-specific bacteria and prevent or eliminate comedones. Too many products and/or measures will be too aggressive and can disrupt the skin barrier. Therefore, the focus is always on mild cleansing and gentle products. It is important to remember that the skin is often irritated and sensitive due to dermatological or cosmetical measures. Both physical and chemical irritation should be avoided in skincare. For this reason, less is often more! To clarify, the steps for an optimal skincare routine are listed below. While one would assume that everyone knows these, practice shows that this is not the case. This list can be printed out and given to patients for their reference.

Skincare Routine Basics

- Do not wash the face with ice-cold water as this will contract the skin pores. Use lukewarm or warm water instead.

- Washing too frequently, especially excessive scrubbing, will aggravate the problem. Don't overdo it! Washing the face gently two or three times a day is enough.

- Avoid soaps with a pH of 8–12 as they disrupt the skin barrier. Soaps also tend to clog the skin pores, so a gentle soap-free cleanser is best.

- Hydrophilic, water-containing products such as light oil in water emulsions are preferable, and ideally hydrogels, which clean without damaging the skin barrier.

- Keep your hands off the pimples. Dirty hands can worsen infections. Also avoid resting your hands or phone against the side of your face.

- Do not manually express pus from pustules. This should only ever be done by a professional with clean equipment and appropriate technique. Non-professional squeezing of pimples can worsen inflammation, resulting in scars and enlarged pores.

- Be careful with exfoliation. Many exfoliating products are too aggressive and damage the skin. When exfoliating, use gentle products, once or twice a week maximum. Consider simply using cloths with a tighter weave, such as a towel or washcloth, for gentle manual exfoliation.

- Do not expose irritated skin to the sun. Aside from the risk of sunburn, particularly for those with sensitive skin, UV radiation primarily hits injured skin and very easily creates hyperpigmentation. Moreover, UV radiation dries out the pimples but it doesn't make them go away. In the long term, it also causes the skin to age more quickly and increases the risk of skin cancer.

- Never go to bed without cleaning the face. All dirt from the course of the day needs to be removed, especially in big cities where pollution is high. Cleanse the face of dirt, bacteria, sweat, and excess sebum before going to sleep.

- Always remove mascara and foundation before going to bed, even when tired. Any make-up residue left behind can clog the skin pores, which can result in more pimples. Cosmetics that are not thoroughly removed can also irritate the skin and eyes.

- Always use a clean towel. Even after a single use, the fabric will pick up many bacteria, which will then transfer to the face if the towel is reused. Therefore, change towels and face cloths very frequently, even daily in acute cases.

Modern Facial Masks Using Chinese Herbs

Chinese herbs that are very commonly used for acne facial masks[7] include *huáng qín* and *dà huáng* for clearing heat; *fú líng* and *jiāng cán* for brightening the skin (used for dark discoloration); *shí gāo*, an option for clearing heat and relieving extreme inflammation often seen in very serious cases of acne rosacea; and *zhēn zhū mǔ*, a very popular choice in many skin problems. *Zhēn zhū mǔ* clears heat and calms the skin.

For application, grind the herbs to a fine powder, mix them together with honey, and apply as a facial mask to the skin. Healing earth would be an alternative if honey is not available. The finely ground herbs would then be mixed with healing earth and dissolved in water before being applied as facial mask. Be flexible!

Cosmetics and Make-Up

Acne-covering measures are helpful psychologically for many patients with both inflammatory acne and post-acne conditions, such as scarring and discoloration. Many acne patients report the positive effect of complexion-correcting measures on their quality of life. The compounds should be well tolerated and easy to use. It goes without saying that patients with acne-prone skin should avoid oily and greasy make-up products, sunscreens, and hair products. As mentioned before, it is important to prevent pores from becoming blocked. The skin must be able to breathe and regenerate. Thus, water-based or non-comedogenic products should be used. A practical hint: It is more and more common that non-comedogenic products will disclose this on their packaging. Therefore, advise patients to pay careful attention to the labels of make-up products.

Make-up utensils should be cleaned regularly. Just as the face should be cleaned regularly, so too should the utensils that are used on the face and neck. One really doesn't want to know what is accumulating in the hairs and fibers of the brushes and sponges with which the patient applies their foundation, powder, or eyeshadow.

Other Skincare Advice: Home Remedies

There are some other applications that have proven useful in practice for many patients. I often advise my patients to use these remedies, as many patients will have these products at home. They are natural and gentle—that's the main thing!

Zinc is a very common home remedy for acne—more precisely, zinc oxide. Small amounts of zinc oxide ointment are applied to the affected skin lesions, and I often recommend it to be used overnight or while at home. It has a disinfectant effect, calms irritated skin, and helps the skin heal. It should be noted that zinc oxide ointment can also have a strong drying effect. Thus, it should not be used for too long—and don't overdo it! Please advise your patients to pay attention to the quality of the product. Many ready-made zinc creams contain a large amount of petroleum jelly. As already mentioned, petroleum jelly is thick and poorly spreadable. It usually leaves a greasy film on the skin and may also clog the pores. Thus, only the affected skin lesions should be covered with a thin layer of the ointment. Again, products vary, so pay attention to the quality of the product.

Aloe vera is another useful home remedy. It has a cooling effect, soothing the skin and relieving redness and itching due to inflammation. Aloe vera generally supports skin regeneration and has a moisturizing effect. Thus, it can also be used in mild cases and for general skincare. When used as a gel, patients should be advised to store the product in the refrigerator because it is very sensitive to oxidation. I often recommend cooling aloe vera taken directly from the fridge when patients have serious acne rosacea. Sometimes, the face is very red and feels hot and inflamed, and using cool aloe vera gives immediate relief.

Healing earth (healing clay) is also very common and easy to use. Healing earth is available as a ready-made paste or as a powder that has to be mixed with water. It is applied to the skin as a mask and left until it is completely dry. The skin is cleaned from dirt, sebum, and bacteria. Clogged pores are released, allowing the skin to be better supplied with nutrients and oxygen. However, please note that healing earth dries out the skin. Patients with sensitive or naturally very dry skin should moisturize the facial skin after treatment.

And last but not least, another home remedy, which everyone will know: **Tea tree oil**. Tea tree oil is a natural essential oil that is extracted from the tea tree. It has an anti-bacterial effect and is applied directly to the inflamed or reddened skin areas for acne treatment. Disadvantages of tea tree oil are that it has a very intense smell and can irritate the skin in sensitive patients. Diluting the oil is thus often recommended. Patients should be advised to pay attention to quality. Similar to other plants, the type of plant, growing conditions, and harvest time can have a major impact on the product.

Endnotes

1 www.ourworldindata.org: Per capita milk consumption, 2017, www.statistica.com: Annual consumption of fluid cow milk worldwide in 2019, by country.

2 Castleman, M. (2009) "The calcium myth." *Natural Solutions*, July/August, 57–62.

3   Most of the information is taken from the book: 张湖德, 张玉苹主编.餐桌上的发物与忌口[M].上海: 上海科学技术出版社. 2007. (Zhang Hu-de, Zhang Yu-ping (chief editors): Fa Wu and Taboos at the Dinner Table [M]. Shanghai Scientific and Technical Publishers).

4   Extracted from *Pǔ Jì Fāng Xīn Biān Tóu Miàn Bù Jí Bìng* (New Version of Pǔ Jì Fāng's Head and Face Diseases). Authors: Guō Zhì-Huá and Xiào Guó-Shì. Beijing: The People's Military Medical Press, 2012. This book is based on the original *Pǔ Jì Fāng*. The authors selected those formulas treating head and facial diseases. They rearranged the order of the formulas and categorized them into head, hair, face, ear, and nose diseases.

5   Míng Dynasty (1368–1644 AD).

6   There were more formulas documented. I have selected three of them.

7   All herbs can be also used as a wash or a wet compress. These applications will be discussed and described in Appendix I.

9

Acne Rosacea
(*Jiǔ Zhā Bí* 酒渣鼻)

ACNE ROSACEA, usually referred to simply as rosacea, is quite often mistaken for acne vulgaris in its early stages. Rosacea is a very common skin disease, which is characterized by redness, papules, pustules, and swelling (of the nose). It is a reoccurring condition, which can be exacerbated by sun exposure, heat, alcohol, strong emotions, caffeine, and spicy foods; however, the exact causes of rosacea have not yet been determined. In Western medicine, there is no cure for rosacea. Some treatments might help but usually only do so for a short period of time.

Unlike acne vulgaris, rosacea is typically localized over the central face—cheeks, nose, forehead, and chin—and does not typically present with comedones. Clinically, rosacea is predominantly identified by an intense reddening of the skin caused by dilation of the superficial vasculature of the face. Patients thus often feel warm in their face.

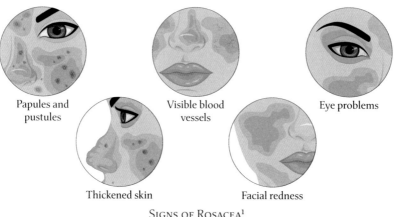

Papules and pustules

Visible blood vessels

Eye problems

Thickened skin

Facial redness

SIGNS OF ROSACEA[1]

Acne Vulgaris vs Acne Rosacea

Acne vulgaris and acne rosacea are characteristically distinct in the ways they affect the skin. It is important to differentiate the two conditions in order to provide the patient with the correct treatment.

	Acne vulgaris	Acne rosacea
Chronic inflammatory disease	Yes	Yes
Common	Yes	Yes
Age of patients	Teenagers and adults	Mostly adults (> 30 years), more women than men
Comedones	Yes	No
Papules and pustules	Yes	Yes (but more serious)
Nodules	Yes	Yes
Areas affected	Widespread (face, back, chest, shoulders)	Central face (flush areas, predominantly nose, forehead, cheeks, chin)
Facial erythema	No	Yes
Rhinophyma[2]	No	Yes[3]
Triggers	Varied (e.g. genetic predisposition, hormonal changes, unhealthy nutrition, stress, cosmetic products, etc.)	Sun, heat, alcohol, strong emotions, caffeine, spicy foods

The Treatment of Acne Rosacea with Chinese Herbal Medicine

For all those who see patients with acne rosacea in practice, I would like to list the three most common TCM syndromes that present in my practice including characteristics, distinguishing features, and correspondent treatment options. This should help you to recognize this complex skin condition in practice and treat it effectively.

Heat Exuberance in the Lung Channel (*Fèi Jīng Rè Shèng Zhèng* 肺经热盛证)
Characteristics

In this pattern, the erythema usually occurs on the tip of the nose or the sides of the nose and blanches when pressed. The skin is warm and feels burning. Papules and pustules are rather rare in this pattern. Accompanying symptoms may include constipation, dark-yellow urine, a dry mouth, and thirst.

The tongue is red with a thin yellow coating. The pulse is rapid and floating, or rapid and slippery if there is phlegm in the Lungs.

Treatment Principle
Clear heat in the Lungs and cool the blood (*qīng fèi rè liáng xuè* 清肺热凉血)

Representative Formula
Pí Pá Qīng Fèi Yĭn (Eriobotrya Decoction to Clear the Lung, also known as Loquat Decoction to Clear the Lung)

Ingredients

pí pá yè	Eriobotryae Japonicae, Folium	15 g
sāng bái pí	Mori, Cortex	12–15 g
huáng băi	Phellodendri, Cortex	9 g
huáng lián	Coptidis, Rhizoma	6 g
rén shēn	Ginseng, Radix	1–3 g
gān căo	Glycyrrhizae Uralensis, Radix	6–9 g

First Reference
This formula originally appeared in the *Wài Kē Dà Chéng* (Great Compendium of External Medicine, 1665), written by Qí Kūn.

Formula Analysis
Please see "Wind-Heat Stagnating in the Lungs" pattern in Chapter 5 for a detailed analysis of this formula.

Modifications
To enhance the heat-clearing and blood-cooling effect, add *Wŭ Wèi Xiāo Dú Yĭn* (Five Ingredient Decoction to Eliminate Toxins). Especially when

the lesions are swollen, particularly those around the nose, and the skin feels burning, hot to the touch, and painful, this formula is very effective. Please see the section "Toxic Heat and Blood Stasis" in Chapter 5 for a detailed explanation of this formula. I also recommend adding herbs such as *mŭ dān pí, chì sháo,* or *dān shēn.* One or two of these in a relatively high dose (10–15 g) are enough to increase the blood-cooling and blood-regulating effect. If the patient is constipated, add *dà huáng* 9 g. For extremely dry mouth and thirst, add *shí gāo* 15 g and *shēng dì huáng* 10–15 g in order to clear heat, cool blood, and nourish yīn. In patients with a long history of rosacea, heat tends to scorch and injure the yīn and body fluids (*jīn yè* 津液) as a consequence. In addition to significant thirst and dryness of the mouth, lips, and throat, the patient may be irritable, restless, and sleepless. As an alternative to the two previously mentioned herbs, one may add *Zhú Yè Shí Gāo Tāng* (Lophatherus and Gypsum Decoction),[4] consisting of *dàn zhú yè* 6–9 g, *shí gāo* 15–30 g, *rén shēn* 3 g, *mài mén dōng* 9–15 g, *zhì bàn xià* 9 g, *jīng mī* 9–12 g, and *zhì gān cǎo* 3–6 g instead. *Zhú Yè Shí Gāo Tāng* is a very good choice when heat affects the Lungs and the Stomach as well, resulting in the symptoms mentioned above. This formula strongly clears heat, generates fluids, and harmonizes the Stomach. It also enhances the flow of qì, which is obstructed due to heat. However, in this pattern I do recommend working with relatively large dosages, whichever composition you choose. The heat seen in this pattern can be extreme and often requires a strong approach to help the patient quickly and effectively. As soon as the skin calms down, one can work more gently by using lower doses, drinking less of the decoction, or starting to slow down the pace by taking a one-day break in between the bags of herbs.

Suggestions for External Treatment

- *Diān Dǎo Sǎn* (Upside Down Powder)

- *Jiĕ Dú Xĭ Gāo* (Detoxifying Lotion)

- *Jiŭ Zhā Bí Gāo* (Rosacea Paste)

Herbal Washes or Wet Compresses

In this pattern, similar herbs and combinations can be used as described in the section "Wind-Heat Stagnating in the Lungs" in Chapter 5. One difference, however, is that I suggest working a little more strongly here. That means using larger dosages, or less water with the same dosages, for greater concentration.

Excellent stand-alone herbs/applications are:

- a facial mask with *shí gāo*

- aloe vera (cold from the fridge).

Example Pictures of the Skin

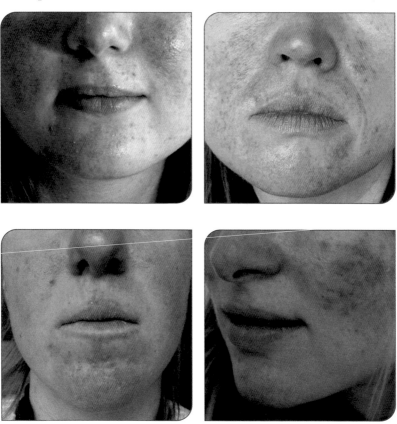

Blood Heat (*Xuè Rè* 血热)

Accumulated heat in the blood is another TCM pattern commonly seen in practice in patients with rosacea. Based on the "four levels" theory developed by Yè Tiān Shì (c. 1667–1746, Qīng Dynasty), which describes the progression of *wēn bìng* (warm and febrile diseases) through the *wèi* (defense), *qì* (qì), *yíng* (nutritive), and *xuè* (blood) levels, in this case heat has reached the blood level or *xuè* level, the deepest level. Thus, the heat is severe, and working gently will not be effective here. Patients have a very high level of suffering and it is better to work strongly and see the patient frequently at the beginning in order to see if, and how quickly, you can help.

Characteristics

At this stage, heat is very severe. The bulb of the nose is dark red, and red papules and pustules surround the nose and the area around the mouth, while small dilated superficial blood vessels, also known as spider veins, occur near the surface of the skin. This phenomenon is called telangiectasias and it is commonly seen on the face in the advanced stages of rosacea, around the nose and cheeks. The skin feels hot and a local burning feeling may be present. Often patients report that the whole face feels warm or hot, and that they love to drink cold drinks and cool the face. However, the greater the heat, the greater the likelihood of it causing blood stasis. The skin lesions will then turn purple and nodules may arise, indicating the need for more blood-moving herbs. Accompanying symptoms can include thirst, dry stools, and dark urination. In women, menstruation may be irregular. It is also quite common, though not essential, that the patient is irritable, restless, and sleepless, as heat is stirring the Heart and the *shén*.

The tongue is red with a yellow coating and the pulse is rapid and wiry or rapid and slippery. Please note that the thicker and more pus-filled the pustules, the more slippery the pulse tends to be.

Treatment Principle

Cool and invigorate blood, clear heat, and relieve toxicity (*liáng xuè huó xuè, qīng rè jiě dú* 凉血活血, 清热解毒).

Representative Formula

Liáng Xuè Sì Wù Tāng (Cool the Blood with Four Substances Decoction), combined with *Huáng Lián Jiě Dú Tāng* (Coptis Decoction to Relieve Toxicity).

Ingredients
Liáng Xuè Sì Wù Tāng (Cool the Blood with Four Substances Decoction)

shēng dì huáng	Rehmanniae Glutinosae, Radix	15–30 g
chì sháo	Paeoniae Rubrae, Radix	10 g
huáng qín	Scutellariae, Radix	10 g
dāng guī	Angelicae Sinensis, Radix	10 g
fú líng	Poriae Cocos, Sclerotium	10 g
hóng huā	Carthami, Flos	10 g
chuān xiōng	Chuanxiong, Rhizoma	10 g
gān căo	Glycyrrhizae Uralensis, Radix	10 g
+/– *shēng jiāng*	Zingiberis Recens, Rhizoma	5 g

Huáng Lián Jiě Dú Tāng (Coptis Decoction to Relieve Toxicity)

huáng lián	Coptidis, Rhizoma	5 g
huáng qín	Scutellariae, Radix	10 g
huáng băi	Phellodendri, Cortex	10 g
zhī zĭ	Gardeniae, Fructus	10 g

First Reference

Liáng Xuè Sì Wù Tāng was first mentioned in the book *Yī Zōng Jīn Jiàn* (The Golden Mirror of Ancestral Medicine, c. 1736–1743), written by Wú Qiān *et al.*

The first reference of *Huáng Lián Jiě Dú Tāng* was in the *Wài Tái Mì Yào* (Arcane Essentials from the Imperial Library, 752), written by Wáng Tāo.

Formula Analysis
Liáng Xuè Sì Wù Tāng

This formula is basically a modification of *Sì Wù Tāng* (Four Substance Decoction). It cools the blood and removes blood stagnation. If the blood-heat aspect is predominant, increase the dosages of the blood-cooling herbs. Conversely, if blood stasis is predominant, it goes without saying that the dosages of the blood-moving herbs should be increased. In detail, *shēng dì huáng* clears heat, cools the blood, and nourishes yīn and blood. *Chì sháo* clears heat, cools the blood, and activates the blood in order to remove blood stagnation. *Huáng qín* drains heat and fire, and fulfills a detoxifying function. *Dāng guī* tonifies blood and invigorates the blood. It reduces swelling, expels pus, generates flesh, and alleviates pain.[5] The pain-reducing effect should not be ignored, as patients often find their skin very painful. *Fú líng* leaches out dampness and harmonizes the middle *jiāo*. *Hóng huā* and *chuān xiōng* invigorate the blood, dispel blood stasis, and relieve pain. *Gān cǎo* clears heat, relieves toxicity, and alleviates pain. It also moderates and harmonizes the properties of other herbs within the formula. Finally, *shēng jiāng* is used to reduce the toxicity of the other herbs or harmonize potential side effects of overdosing the other herbs. As it can warm the middle *jiāo*, it can protect the "middle" from the many cold herbs within the formula.

Huáng Lián Jiě Dú Tāng
Please see the section "Toxic Heat (*Rè Dú Zhèng* 热毒证)" in Chapter 5 for detailed analysis of this formula and description of herb actions.

Modifications

If there is excessive secretion of sebum and the skin looks very oily, add *shān zhā* and *zé xiè* 12–15 g of each herb. In case of severe papules and pustules filled with pus, add *Wǔ Wèi Xiāo Dú Yǐn* (Five Ingredient Decoction to Eliminate Toxins) or *tǔ fú líng* 15–30 g. One may add *bái huā shé shé cǎo* 10–15 g if the areas of erythema are enlarged, obviously swollen, hot, and painful, as it strongly clears heat and resolves toxicity. If the patient is constipated, add *dà huáng* 10 g.

To conclude this pattern, I would like to mention an herbal prescription that is often given as a medicinal tea. However, I would like to recommend it as a conventional herbal tea for severe cases of rosacea. Patients can drink the tea throughout the day in addition to their normal drinks. The herbs can be boiled as a normal decoction but with more water to make it suitable for drinking as a regular tea. It can also be brewed with hot water like any other flower tea. The mixture can be brewed several times. The formula is called *Liáng Xuè Wǔ Huā Tāng* (Cool the Blood Decoction with Five Flowers) consisting of:

hóng huā	Carthami, Flos	10 g
jī guān huā	Celosiae Cristata, Flos	10 g
líng xiāo huā	Campsis, Flos	10 g
méi guī huā	Rosae Rugosae, Flos	10 g
yě jú huā	Chrysanthemi Indici, Flos	10 g

This herbal combination can clear heat and cool the blood. It is often seen in the treatment of acne rosacea in the blood heat pattern, although I think it is too weak as a stand-alone formula. It can be a perfect addition to the standard herbal treatment with TCM, especially in cases with severe erythema and extreme redness of the bulb of the nose.

Suggestions for External Treatment

- *Diān Dǎo Sǎn* (Upside Down Powder)

- *Huà Dú Sǎn Gāo* (Toxicity Transforming Powder Paste)

- *Jiě Dú Xǐ Gāo* (Detoxifying Lotion)

- *Jiǔ Zhā Bí Gāo* (Rosacea Paste)

- *San Huáng Xǐ Jì* (Three Yellow Cleanser Formula)

- *Sì Huáng Gāo* (Four Yellow Paste)

- *Zǐ Yún Gāo* (Purple Cloud Ointment)[6]

Herbal Washes or Wet Compresses
In this pattern, similar herbs and combinations can be used as for the "Toxic Heat and Blood Stasis" pattern, described in detail in Chapter 5. Don't forget that herbs can be added or taken out any time. Be flexible!

The following gives very good results in practice:

- a facial mask with *shí gāo*

- followed with aloe vera (cold from the fridge) to soothe the skin.

Example Pictures of the Skin

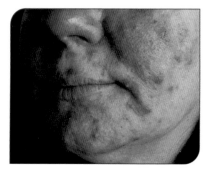
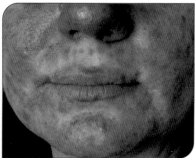
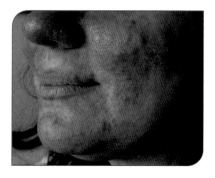

Qì Stagnation and Blood Stasis (*Qì Zhì Xuè Yū* 气滞血瘀)

This pattern is commonly seen if rosacea is left untreated. The main and distinguishing characteristic of this pattern is the knobby bumps on the nose, which make the nose appear swollen. This condition is called rhinophyma, a bulbous nose that is colloquially called "cauliflower nose."

Characteristics

This pattern is characterized by a large, dark-red or purple, bumpy nose. Pores are enlarged and, as in the previous pattern, spider veins can be observed. The skin on the face is generally darker red and purple than in the previous patterns, because stasis is predominant here. Accompanying symptoms may include irregular and painful menstruation with dark blood and clotting.

The tongue has a livid (purple or dark) discoloration and/or purplish veins underneath the tongue, or stasis spots. The deeper the blood stagnation, the more signs can be observed. The pulse can be wiry or rough.

Treatment Principle

Invigorate blood, dispel blood stasis, soften masses and dissipate nodules (*huó xuè qū yū, xiāo zhǒng sàn jié* 活血祛瘀, 消肿散结).

Representative Formula

Tōng Qiào Huó Xuè Tāng (Unblock the Orifices and Invigorate the Blood Decoction) with modifications.

Ingredients

táo rén	Persicae, Semen	10 g
hóng huā	Carthami, Flos	10 g
chuān xiōng	Chuanxiong, Rhizoma	6–10 g
dāng guī	Angelicae Sinensis, Radix	10 g
chì sháo	Paeoniae Rubrae, Radix	10 g
shēng dì huáng	Rehmanniae Glutinosae, Radix	10–12 g
mǔ dān pí	Moutan, Cortex	10 g
xià kū cǎo	Prunellae Vulgaris, Spica	10 g
yě jú huā	Chrysanthemi Indici, Flos	10 g
líng xiāo huā	Campsis, Flos	3–6 g
gān cǎo	Glycyrrhizae Uralensis, Radix	6 g

The original formula contains:

chì sháo	Paeoniae Rubrae, Radix	3 g
chuān xiōng	Chuanxiong, Rhizoma	3 g
táo rén	Persicae, Semen	9 g
hóng huā	Carthami, Flos	9 g
shè xiāng[7]	Moschus	0.15 g
shēng jiāng	Zingiberis Recens, Rhizoma	9 g
cōng bái[8]	Allii Fistulosi, Bulbus	3 g
dà zǎo	Jujubae, Fructus	7 pieces

Add a small amount of white wine, 250 ml, to the decoction.

First Reference

The first reference of *Tōng Qiào Huó Xuè Tāng* was in the *Yī Lín Gǎi Cuò* (Corrections of Errors Among Physicians, 1830), written by Wáng Qīng-Rèn.

Formula Analysis

This formula is basically a modification of *Xuè Fǔ Zhú Yū Tāng* (Drive Out Stasis in the Mansion of Blood Decoction).[9] The main effect of this formula is to stimulate blood circulation and to remove blood stagnation in the head and face area. This formula is commonly used for various disorders characterized by stagnation of blood in the head and face, such as rosacea, headaches, tinnitus, or, in severe cases, even stroke. However, in the treatment of rosacea, it must be modified in order to achieve the desired effect. To make the difference between the ingredients in the modified and original formula clear, I have also listed the original formula above. The modified version used in treating rosacea is analyzed below.

In this formula, *táo rén* and *hóng huā* invigorate blood and break up blood stasis. *Chuān xiōng* invigorates blood and promotes the movement of qì. Always keep in mind, "If the qì circulates, then the blood will circulate."[10] *Dāng guī* and *chì sháo* invigorate the blood, whereas *dāng guī* also nourishes blood and moistens dryness, and *chì sháo* can also cool the blood and clear heat. Combined with *shēng dì huáng*, which cools blood, clears heat, and boosts yīn, the formula is able to dispel blood stasis but nourish and protect blood and yīn while eliminating heat. *Mǔ dān pí* in addition boosts the heat-clearing and blood-cooling effect without injuring the blood or yīn. Please note that unprocessed *mǔ dān pí* effectively clears blood heat, but it can easily harm the stomach. Particularly in cases of long-term use of this herb, (*chǎo*) *mǔ dān pí* (dry-fried) is advisable, because the cold property has been reduced, but the blood heat-clearing effect is still ensured. Thus, it is more tolerable for the digestive system. *Xià kū cǎo* cools heat and dissipates nodules[11] and is particularly effective when qì stagnation has transformed into heat or fire. Similarly, be mindful of patients with a weak Spleen and Stomach, and don't use this herb long-term. *Yě jú huā* clears heat and resolves toxicity, and is particularly effective when the skin feels hot and is painful and swollen. In combination with *xià kū cǎo*, this effect is enhanced. Furthermore, be attentive because rosacea can also affect the eyes in some cases, which is called "ocular rosacea." This condition is often overlooked. The symptoms are generally dry, irritated, swollen, or red eyes. For this, *yě jú huā* and *xià kū cǎo* provide perfect relief when used together. Always remember that flowers are excellent for treating skin conditions on the face. They are light in weight and thus can rise to the head/face. *Líng xiāo huā*, for example, breaks up blood stasis and also cools the blood. In practice, it is often used when women have menstrual problems in addition to their skin issues, such as irregular menstruation or amenorrhea combined with stress or emotional tension. Finally, *gān căo* harmonizes the prescription because it mediates the extreme properties of the other herbs.

Comment: Some might think that *Táo Hóng Si Wù Tāng* (Four Substance Decoction with Safflower and Peach Kernel) or *Hăi Zăo Yù Hú Tāng* (Sargassum Decoction for the Jade Flask) can or should be used in the treatment of this pattern. That is really a matter of personal preference. I don't recommend using any of these formulas because they would require so many modifications that one arrives at the above-mentioned formula in any case.

Modifications

For pustules, add *Wŭ Wèi Xiāo Dú Yĭn* (Five Ingredient Decoction to Eliminate Toxins). For severe erythema with skin that is burning and feels hot and painful, add *bái huā shé shé căo* with a dosage of at least 15 g. *Zăo xiū* 10 g can also be added. It is very effective in draining heat, relieving fire toxicity, and reducing swelling and inflammation of the affected skin lesions. It enhances skin healing and can reduce the pain of lesions. For irregular and painful menstruation with dark blood and clotting, add *yì mŭ căo* 10–12 g and *yán hú suŏ* 10–12 g. If the blood stasis is combined with phlegm, one may add *Hăi Zăo Yù Hú Tāng* in order to transform phlegm and soften hardness. *Hăi Zăo Yù Hú Tāng* is analyzed in detail in the section "Knotting Together of Phlegm and Blood Stasis" in Chapter 5. Finally, for patients with a weak digestion, add (*shēng*) *yì yĭ rén* 10–12 g. (*Shēng*) *yì yĭ rén* protects the Spleen and it can cool heat. An alternative is *bái zhú* 10 g.

Suggestions for External Treatment

- *Diān Dăo Săn* (Upside Down Powder)

- *Hēi Bù Yào Gāo* (Black Cloth Medicated Paste)[12]

- *Hóng Huā Gāo* (Safflower Ointment)

- *Jiŭ Zhā Bí Gāo* (Rosacea Paste)

- *Sì Huáng Gāo* (Four Yellow Paste)

Herbal Washes or Wet Compresses

Frequently used and effective herbs for external washes in this pattern are: *táo rén, hóng huā, dān shēn, zào jiǎo cì, sān qī, pú gōng yīng, gān cǎo, lián qiáo, jīn yín huā, zhāng nǎo, dú huó, dà huáng,* or *xià kū cǎo.* As already mentioned, the variety of options of Chinese herbs for external treatment are nearly endless. Herbs are chosen according to their action to promote blood circulation, remove blood, soften nodules, and ease pain. However, be flexible—if more heat-clearing action is needed, increase herbs such as *pú gōng yīng* or *dà huáng.* You can also add herbs such as *bái huā shé shé cǎo* to maximize the heat-cooling and toxicity-resolving action. As always, a maximum of three to four herbs in combination is enough. Let me give you some simple examples:

sān qī	Notoginseng, Radix	10 g
dà huáng	Rhei, Radix et Rhizoma	10 g
xià kū cǎo	Prunellae Vulgaris, Spica	15 g

sān qī	Notoginseng, Radix	15 g
dú huó	Angelicae Pubescentis, Radix	10 g
zhāng nǎo	Camphora	5 g

These combinations are suitable for 250–300 ml of water.

dān shēn	Salviae Miltiorhizae, Radix	15 g
gān cǎo	Glycyrrhizae Uralensis, Radix	10 g
dà huáng	Rhei, Radix et Rhizoma	10 g
or *bái huā shé shé cǎo*	Hedyotis Diffusae, Herba	15 g

Suitable for 300 ml of water.

Example Pictures of the Skin[13]

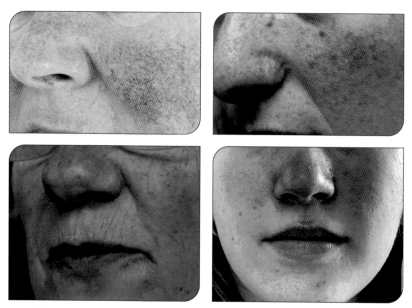

Please note these are relatively mild stages of this pattern. The color of the skin clearly shows blood stasis due to its slightly purplish coloration.

Useful Advice About the Course and Prognosis of Treatment

For rosacea, it is crucial to inform your patient about the duration of treatment. Rosacea has already become chronic in most of the cases we see in practice. Thus, a realistic benchmark you can promise your patients is a minimum of six months of treatment with Chinese herbal medicine. However, the first goal should be to reduce the erythema and alleviate the pain on the skin, which will give your patients initial encouragement as they continue their treatment. Many patients with rosacea tell me that they are often asked about their skin prior to treatment. Over the course of the treatment, they report how happy they are when others no longer question them or look at them strangely. This is already a success from a psychological point of view.

Preventive Healthcare: Dietary, Lifestyle, and Skincare Advice

The diet, lifestyle, and skincare advice for patients with rosacea is very similar to that described for acne in Chapter 8. However, extra emphasis is placed on avoiding too much coffee, red wine and spirits, sugar, fried and deep-fried dishes, as well as curries, chili, and any other hot spices. Patients with rosacea should avoid food and drinks that bring heat to the inside or aggravate already existing heat in any case. Moreover, they should avoid heat and sun exposure. This is simple advice but very important. The use of a light-textured sunscreen with a high sun protection factor is strongly recommended as well.

Endnotes

1   Source: Shutterstock.

2   Enlargement of the nose.

3   Not all patients will have rhinophyma.

4   Also known as "Bamboo Leaves and Gypsum Combination" or "Decoction of Bamboo Leaf and Gypsum."

5   Bensky, D., Clavey, S., and Stöger, E. (2004) *Materia Medica*, 3rd edition. Seattle, WA: Eastland Press, p.751.

6   May contain herbs that are restricted or forbidden in some countries.

7   *Shè xiāng* comes from an endangered animal species and is thus forbidden in many countries these days. Most Chinese medicinal products no longer contain it, or it is replaced by medicines with a similar mode of action.

8   This herb is also called *lǎo cōng* (老葱).

9   *Xuè Fǔ Zhú Yū Tāng: táo rén, hóng huā, dāng guī, chuān xiōng, chì sháo, niú xī, chái hú, jié gěng, zhǐ ké, shēng dì huáng, gān cǎo.*

10 Scheid, V., Bensky, D., Ellis, A., and Barolet, R. (2009) *Formulas and Strategies*, 2nd edition. Seattle, WA: Eastland Press, p.565.

11 Bensky, D., Clavey, S., and Stöger, E. (2004) *Materia Medica*, 3rd edition. Seattle, WA: Eastland Press, p.102.

12 May contain herbs that are restricted or forbidden in some countries.

13 Source of the first two pictures: Shutterstock.

11

Clinical Cases of Acne and Rosacea

I N THIS CHAPTER, five case studies of acne and one case of rosacea are presented to showcase how Chinese herbal medicine is applied in clinical practice, and to demonstrate how the patient's skin improves over the course of treatment. This will give you a deeper understanding of the use of Chinese herbs, and increase your confidence in prescribing them to your patients in your own practice.

If you look closely at the individual herbal formulas, you will recognize that many of them are based on classical formulas, with the addition of several herbal combinations that are used again and again because of their known efficacy. The ability to prescribe the correct base formula and flexibly modify it to fit the individual case is one of the central skills of an experienced TCM practitioner and the key to selecting the right herbal prescription.

#1: Female Patient, 22 Years Old–Acne
First Visit

This young woman presented in the clinic with facial acne on her cheeks and around her nose that had been present for nearly one year. Her skin was red and felt warm. The acne manifested as bright-red, inflamed papules, occasionally pustules, which were painful and sometimes itchy. The skin on her upper arms showed the small bumps of "keratosis pilaris."[1] She was a very stressed young woman, currently studying and under a lot of pressure, much of it self-directed. Sometimes she felt a sensation of internal heat, especially in times of strain and overload. She also complained of occasional constipation; otherwise, her eating patterns and digestion were normal. Her menstrual cycle was also normal, with no irregularity or pain.

She had a thin and small tongue, with redness at the tip. The pulse was rapid and weak.

TCM Diagnosis

Wind-Heat Stagnating in the Lungs (*Fēng Rè Fàn Fèi Zhèng* 风热犯肺证).

Treatment Principle

Clear heat in the Lungs and dispel wind (*qīng fèi qū fēng* 清肺祛风).

Formula

Modified *Pí Pá Qīng Fèi Yǐn* (Eriobotrya Decoction to Clear the Lung):

pí pá yè	Eriobotryae Japonicae, Folium	12 g
sāng bái pí	Mori, Cortex	12 g
huáng qín	Scutellariae, Radix	12 g
yú xīng cǎo	Houttuynia Cordata Thunb., Herba	30 g
pú gōng yīng	Taraxaci, Herba	30 g
zǐ huā dì dīng	Violae, Herba	30 g
zhè bèi mǔ	Fritillariae Thunbergii, Bulbus	15 g
dān shēn	Salviae Miltiorhizae, Radix	15 g
xià kū cǎo	Prunellae Vulgaris, Spica	12 g
zào jiǎo cì	Gleditsiae, Spina	12 g
jiǎo gǔ lán	Gynostemma Pentaphyllum, Herba	12 g

Raw herbs taken as a decoction, twice daily for 10–14 days.

Case Analysis

This case of acne is a typical result of wind-heat invasion of the Lungs. The pathogenic wind-heat ascends to the head, giving rise to facial acne. Heat consumes the body fluids, resulting in dryness. Keratosis pilaris on the patient's upper arms is a good indicator for dryness of the skin. A thin and small tongue can indicate that either yīn or qì is deficient. Wind-heat may injure the Lung yīn, but Lung yīn deficiency can also result from longer-lasting Lung qì deficiency. One can view it from different directions. However, signs of heat and dryness were the predominant characteristics in this case, and we as practitioners treat what we see. The red tip of the tongue is a sign of wind-heat, and her rapid pulse also indicates heat. The fact that her pulse was weak was a reflection of her weak and deficient general constitution. Note that the pulse in the wind-heat pattern is often superficial. In this case, it was not. However, all other signs spoke for themselves.

The formula given to this patient was based on modified *Pí Pá Qīng Fèi Yǐn* (Eriobotrya Decoction to Clear the Lung) with the chief herbs *pí pá yè* and *sāng bái pí*. *Huáng qín* was added to enhance the heat-clearing effects of the formula, especially in the upper *jiāo*. Combined with *sāng bái pí*, it is effective in clearing heat from the Lungs, in both acute and chronic conditions. *Yú xīng cǎo* is very frequently used to treat acne as it disperses heat and resolves toxicity, and acts especially on the Lungs.[2] Combined with *pú gōng yīng*, it is very effective in clearing heat and treating inflamed acne lesions. Both *yú xīng cǎo* and *pú gōng yīng* can be used in relatively high dosages of 30 g as seen in this case, but as soon as the desired effect is reached, the dosage can be reduced. As with all cooling herbs, use them with caution in weak patients and in those with a weak digestion. It may have been observed that part of the formula *Wǔ Wèi Xiāo Dú Yǐn* (Five Ingredient Decoction to Eliminate Toxins) was incorporated into this prescription, namely *pú gōng yīng* and *zǐ huā dì dīng*. Both of these herbs can strongly clear heat and resolve toxicity, while *zǐ huā dì dīng* also cools the blood and reduces swellings.[3] *Zhè bèi mǔ*, cold in nature and bitter in taste, was used for its ability to drain heat and transform phlegm-heat. *Xià kū cǎo* was added to this formula. In combination with *zhè bèi mǔ*, it can reduce painful swellings and it is good for Lung heat patterns with productive cough (thick yellow sputum).[4] In this case, it was used to soothe and alleviate the inflamed acne lesions. *Dān shēn* was used to cool and regulate the blood, and to prevent blood stasis. As a reminder, the more dark-red, purplish, hard, and painful the acne lesions are, the more herbs that cool and regulate the blood are needed. Finally, *zào jiǎo cì* is useful for blind pimples, as it opens the skin pores to allow the contents of the pimples to drain. In addition, it can also invigorate blood. The reason for prescribing *jiǎo gǔ lán* was that the patient had a weak constitution. *Jiǎo gǔ lán* tonifies qì, strengthening endurance and lessening the effect of fatigue, as well as strengthening the patient's immunity, and it is often used in patients with a poor constitution and weak immune system.[5]

Second Visit

After 14 days, the skin had become less red and warm. The acne lesions were reduced and less inflamed and painful. The patient's stools were more regular, but at this visit she reported delayed menstruation with a bit less blood than her normal flow, compared with before starting the herbs.

Formula Modification

The dosage of *yú xīng cǎo*, *pú gōng yīng*, and *zǐ huā dì dīng* was reduced to 15 g of each herb. *Yì mǔ cǎo* 12 g was added and the patient was informed to stop taking the herbs shortly before her next period, because the intake of too many cooling herbs tends to block the menstrual flow. Although not always the case, sometimes this can be quite a simple explanation when a woman reports that her period is delayed and scanty while taking herbs for treating the skin. In such a case, either stop the formula shortly before the period is due and/or add herbs such as *yì mǔ cǎo* to improve the menstrual flow.

Clinical Course

After taking herbs for another three weeks, there were fewer papules, and the skin was no longer painful and itchy. The patient was advised to continue the herbs for another four weeks, or for longer if her skin still had any discomfort. She was reminded about the importance of reducing stress and maintaining a healthy diet.

Practical hint on keratosis pilaris: You may advise your patients to massage the affected skin areas gently with a soft brush. This creates an exfoliating effect to remove the dry skin scales, but also improves blood circulation. When blood can circulate freely, it can nourish the skin.

#2: Female Patient, 25 Years Old–Acne

This young female patient presented in the clinic with facial acne, mainly on the cheeks. The acne manifested as deep, inflamed papules and pustules that were painful with pressure. Her skin appearance tended to worsen before her menstrual period. Besides symptoms of bloating, slightly softer stools, breast distension, and mood changes before her period, no other symptoms were reported.

The color of the tongue was pale and slightly purplish. The tongue was thick with tooth-marks. Her pulse was wiry and slightly slippery.

TCM Diagnosis

Liver Depression Transforms into Heat and Spleen Deficiency (*gān yù huà rè, pí xū* 肝郁化热, 脾虚).

Treatment Principle

Clear Liver heat and drain fire, rectify qì, and fortify the Spleen (*qīng gān xiè huǒ, lǐ qì jiàn pí* 清肝泻火, 理气健脾).

Formula

(*chǎo*) *huáng qín*	Scutellariae, Radix (dry-fried)	9 g
(*chǎo*) *mǔ dān pí*	Moutan, Cortex (dry-fried)	12 g
pú gōng yīng	Taraxaci, Herba	15 g
dài dài huā	Citri Aurantii Amarae, Flos	3 g
líng xiāo huā	Campsis, Flos	3 g
hóng huā	Carthami, Flos	3 g
yú xīng cǎo	Houttuynia Cordata Thunb., Herba	15 g
zào jiǎo cì	Gleditsiae, Spina	6 g
bái zhú	Atractylodis Macrocephalae, Rhizoma	9 g
sāng bái pí	Mori, Cortex	10 g
lǜ è méi	Armeniacae Mume, Flos	3 g
méi guī huā	Rosae Rugosae, Flos	3 g

Raw herbs taken as a decoction, twice daily for 14 days.

Case Analysis

In this case, the patient's tongue and pulse, combined with the skin appearance, was sufficient to make a precise diagnosis. A good practitioner should be able to accurately assess just a few signs in order to design a beneficial treatment strategy. One may note that many flowers were used within the formula. The young woman reported mood changes before her period, but it was obvious that there were other factors causing her stress, although she didn't discuss them. As mentioned previously, flowers should be considered for the treatment of any skin condition on the face as they are light in weight and thus can rise to the face while regulating qì and calming emotions.

All emotional aspects are very important in treating patients with skin conditions on the face such as acne. The most suitable flowers to incorporate are: *líng xiāo huā*, *lǜ è méi*, *hé huān huā*, *dài dài huā*, *méi guī huā*, or *yě jú huā*. In this particular case, *líng xiāo huā*, *lǜ è méi*, *dài dài huā*, and *méi guī huā* were given. However, the main treatment strategy was to clear Liver heat and drain fire because of the deep inflamed nature of the acne, and its exacerbation premenstrually. For this, *huáng qín* and *mǔ dān pí* were the key herbs. *Huáng qín* has been used in its prepared form *chǎo* (dry-fried) to moderate its bitter and cool nature in order to protect the Spleen and Stomach. The same applies for *mǔ dān pí*, which was also used as (*chǎo*) *mǔ dān pí* for this reason. There are many other useful herbal combinations to be found in this formula. For example, *huáng qín* combined with *pú gōng yīng* is an effective herbal combination to clear heat and resolve toxicity, actions that are needed in order to relieve the inflamed and painful papules and pustules on the patient's face. *Líng xiāo huā*, *hóng huā*, and *zào jiǎo cì* dispel blood stasis, and the combination of *líng xiāo huā* and *zào jiǎo cì* can also cool the blood and draw out toxicity. Relatively small dosages of these three herbs are sufficient. In contrast, a higher dosage of *yú xīng cǎo* was applied in this case. It has a strong action on clearing away heat and toxin, and reducing swellings. The use of *yú xīng cǎo* can be seen in many prescriptions in the treatment of acne. It can be also used as a stand-alone herb for the external treatment of acne, as a wet compress.[6] It is effective and very affordable, and only needs to be applied for 15 minutes once or twice a day. The treatment principle also includes "rectify qì and fortify the Spleen." For this, *bái zhú* was given, in order to strengthen the Spleen and enhance its transportive and transformative function.

Second Visit

The young female patient returned to the clinic two weeks later. The acne lesions had begun to decrease a little and the inflammation had slowly receded. Her tongue was less purplish in color, and she reported that the pimples were less painful.

Formula Modification

As her next period was approaching, *chái hú* 9 g, (*chǎo*) *zhǐ ké* 6 g, and (*chǎo*) *zhī zǐ* 9 g were added. *Chái hú* and (*chǎo*) *zhǐ ké* promote the flow of qì and are based on the formula *Chái Hú Shū Gān Sǎn* (Bupleurum Powder to Spread the Liver). They were given to improve the premenstrual bloating, breast distension, and mood changes. *Zhī zǐ*, in particular, is frequently given if moods tend to be irritated and nervous. If the patient was depressed or introverted, this herb would be not the right choice. *Zhī zǐ* was given in its prepared *chǎo* (dry-fried) form to protect the digestive system while still being effective at clearing heat. The patient was advised to continue taking the herbs for another three weeks.

Clinical Course

After another three weeks, the pimples were significantly reduced. There were hardly any deep pimples now, and those that had previously been inflamed had started to heal. It was important at this time to support skin healing in order to prevent dark lesions and scarring later on. Thus, *dān shēn* 15 g and *zǎo xiū* 3 g were added to the already modified prescription to promote blood circulation and the healing process of the skin. The patient reported that premenstrual signs were much less pronounced. The bloating and breast distension were reduced, and her stools were more normal before and at the start of her period. However, the patient was advised to take the herbs for another month and to come back to the clinic if her skin got worse again or with any other new complaints. Additionally, the patient was informed about the importance of regular exercise in order to move her qì and maintain a stable mood. Interestingly, this has to be repeated in clinic again and again. And patients often confirm that it is good for them to hear this again even though they are aware of it deep inside. Sometimes this information is just too well hidden, buried deeply because everything else seems to be more important for them.

#3: Female Patient, 27 Years Old–Acne

First Visit

This young woman of obese stature presented with acne mainly around her mouth and on her forehead. The acne appeared as deep and dark pimples, particularly those around the mouth. Her forehead was almost covered with dark-red and purplish pustules and nodules, which were painful on pressure and itchy. Her forehead showed increased sebum production, with shining oily skin. Her face also tended to turn red quickly. Examination with the transillumination light lamp[7] confirmed a slight bacterial skin infection.

Accompanying symptoms included fatigue, poor appetite, especially in the morning, easily feeling full after eating, and loose stools.

Her tongue was puffy with a thick coating. The pulse was slippery and smooth.

TCM Diagnosis

Internal Accumulation of Phlegm and Dampness and Blood Stagnation (*tán shī zǔ nèi jiān yū xuè* 痰湿阻内兼瘀血).

Treatment Principle

Eliminate dampness and resolve phlegm, activate blood circulation, and resolve nodules (*qū shī huà tán, huó xuè xiāo zhēng* 祛湿化痰, 活血消癥).

Formula

pí pá yè	Eriobotryae Japonicae, Folium	30 g
sāng bái pí	Mori, Cortex	20 g
(zhú lì) bàn xià	Pinelliae, Rhizoma (prepared in bamboo juice)	9 g
fú líng	Poriae Cocos, Sclerotium	12 g
(chǎo) bái biǎn dòu	Lablab Album, Semen (dry-fried)	12 g
yì yǐ rén	Coices, Semen	30 g
chén pí	Citri Reticulatae, Pericarpium	10 g
zào jiǎo cì	Gleditsiae, Spina	12 g
bái zhǐ	Angelica Dahuricae, Radix	9 g
bái huā shé shé cǎo	Hedyotis Diffusae, Herba	15 g
dà fù pí	Arecae, Pericarpium	9 g

Raw herbs taken as a decoction, twice daily for 12 days.

Case Analysis

This case of acne was caused by phlegm and dampness binding together with blood stasis. The prescription in the treatment of this young woman was mainly based on the modified formulas *Pí Pá Qīng Fèi Yǐn* (Eriobotrya

Decoction to Clear the Lung) and *Èr Chén Tāng* (Decoction of Two Old (Cured) Drugs). While *Èr Chén Tāng* primarily treats phlegm and damp, *Pí Pá Qīng Fèi Yǐn* is used to treat heat and eliminate inflammation. Keep in mind that long-term dampness always tends to generate heat and, later, fire, the more severe form of heat. This can be seen here in the very dark color of the lesions and the recurring flushes on the patient's face. However, clinical experience shows that pimples around the mouth are more difficult to treat than pimples on the forehead. In general, this case was not an easy treatment considering the location and severity of the patient's acne. The key herbs for draining heat downwards, especially heat in the Lungs and resolving phlegm, were *pí pá yè* and *sāng bái pí*. *Bàn xià*, *fú líng*, *bái biǎn dòu*, *yì yǐ rén*, *chén pí*, and *dà fù pí* in combination dry dampness, transform phlegm, and regulate and harmonize the middle *jiāo*. *Bàn xià* was prepared in bamboo juice, which is then called (*zhú lì*) *bàn xià*. When processed in this way, *bàn xià* is more cooling, its drying property is slightly reduced, and its phlegm-resolving action is enhanced, making it more effective in treating phlegm that is combined with heat. *Bái biǎn dòu* was dry-fried (*chǎo*) because this method of preparation enhances the herb's ability to tonify the Spleen, transform dampness, and harmonize the middle *jiāo*.[8] *Zào jiǎo cì* and *bái zhǐ* were both used to bring out sebum or pus from the deep pimples that do not open. Thus, both herbs help detoxify in order to relieve swelling. In addition, *zào jiǎo cì* invigorates the blood. For this reason, it was used in a relatively large dosage of 12 g. *Bái huā shé shé cǎo* was added to increase the anti-inflammatory effects. It strongly clears heat and resolves toxicity, and is often used when thick, red, and painful pustules filled with pus are predominant.

Second Visit

The patient returned two weeks later. The acne lesions had started to lessen, and the color of the pimples hd begun to fade. The pain on pressure and the itching was also slightly reduced. Moreover, her forehead appeared less oily. Her pulse had also become less slippery than when she began treatment.

Formula Modification

Pí pá yè was reduced to 20 g, *sāng bái pí* to 12 g, *yì yǐ rén* to 15 g, and *bái huā shé shé cǎo* to 12 g. The patient was told to continue taking the herbs for at least another four weeks.

Clinical Course

Five weeks after the second consultation, the pimples around her mouth and on her forehead had significantly reduced. The color of the acne had now obviously faded. However, the young patient was told that further improvements in the color would take time, as many of the lesions had been there for a very long time and were deep. She was advised to take better care with her skincare routine and her eating habits from now on. Dairy should be strictly avoided, and she should use as little make-up as possible to cover the acne. Gentle cleansing was recommended, and she should never forget to wash her face before going to bed. It turned out that she had been a bit too nonchalant with all of this in the past. She reported feeling more energetic and her digestion continued to improve. *Bái huā shé shé cǎo* was removed from the herbal formula, *zào jiǎo cì* was reduced to 9 g, and *dān shēn* 9 g, *yì mǔ cǎo* 15 g, and *méi guī huā* 3 g were added. *Dān shēn* and *yì mǔ cǎo* were added to enhance the blood-moving function, and *méi guī huā* to bring the formula to the face.

#4: Female Patient, 27 Years Old–Acne
First Visit

This young woman presented with very severe acne all over her face. The acne manifested as deep and dark-red pustules varying in size, inflamed, and filled with pus, thus also painful. The patient's skin already showed a lot of scarring as she had been experiencing acne for a long time. Both her facial skin and her hair appeared oily, and her appearance in general looked a bit unkempt. After questioning, she affirmed that she liked to eat spicy food and often consumed fast food. She had a slightly foul taste in her mouth as well as bad breath, and also tended to get constipated.

Her tongue was red with a thick yellow greasy coating. Her pulse was rapid and slightly slippery.

TCM Diagnosis

Accumulation of Dampness-Heat in the Body (*shī rè yùn jié* 湿热蕴结).

Treatment Principle

Clear heat and drain dampness (*qīng rè lì shī* 清热利湿).

Formula

yīn chén hāo	Artemisiae Scopariae, Herba	15 g
mǔ dān pí	Moutan, Cortex	12 g
gān cǎo	Glycyrrhizae Uralensis, Radix	6 g
zhè bèi mǔ	Fritillariae Thunbergii, Bulbus	15 g
yì yǐ rén	Coices, Semen	30 g
shí chāng pú	Acori Tatarinowii, Rhizoma	9 g
shí gāo	Gypsum Fibrosum	30 g
zhī mǔ	Anemarrhenae, Rhizoma	6 g
yù zhú	Polygonati Odorati, Rhizoma	9 g
qīng hāo	Artemisiae Annuae, Herba	6g
bái huā shé shé cǎo	Hedyotis Diffusae, Herba	6 g
dà fù pí	Arecae, Pericarpium	6 g
chái hú	Bupleuri, Radix	9 g
yú xīng cǎo	Houttuynia Cordata Thunb., Herba	15 g
dàn zhú yè	Lophatheri, Herba	9 g
zào jiǎo cì	Gleditsiae, Spina	6 g

Raw herbs taken as a decoction, twice daily for 12 days.

Case Analysis

The main treatment strategy for this patient was to clear heat and drain dampness. The prescription can be divided into several herbal groups that fulfill different actions and are often used together in formulas. *Yīn chén hāo* and *qīng hāo* are both aromatic and resolve damp-heat. *Gān cǎo*, *zhè bèi mǔ*, and *yì yǐ rén* clear heat, expel pus, and expel damp-heat. Due to their detoxifying effect, they help reduce skin inflammation, swelling, and pain. *Shí chāng pú* transforms dampness, strengthens the Spleen, and promotes the movement of qì.[9] *Dà fù pí* has similar actions. However, *shí gāo*, *zhī mǔ*, and *dàn zhú yè* clear heat and drain fire. *Shí gāo* and *zhī mǔ* are used in *Bái Hǔ Tāng* (White Tiger Decoction), and *dàn zhú yè* plus *shí gāo* in *Zhú Yè Shí Gāo Tāng* (Lophatherus and Gypsum Decoction).[10] *Yù zhú* nourishes the yīn and clears heat from the Lungs and the Stomach. This yīn-nourishing quality is particularly useful when heat and fire are purged at the same time in the treatment, as it prevents potential harm to the yīn. *Bái huā shé shé cǎo* was used for its inflammation-reducing effects. It strongly clears heat and resolves toxicity and helps to resolve the thick and painful lesions filled with pus. *Chái hú* is bitter, acrid, and cool. It relieves qì constraint by restoring the normal flow of qì and clearing constrained heat. As seen in many other acne formulas, *yú xīng cǎo* was used because it can disperse heat and resolve toxicity. *Zào jiǎo cì* relieves toxicity, discharges pus from stubborn closed pimples, and invigorates the blood. Similarly, *mǔ dān pí* not only strongly clears heat and cools the blood, but it also invigorates blood. Please keep in mind that the qì- and blood-moving aspect is also necessary in order to prevent stasis.

Second Visit

The patient returned for her follow-up consultation about two weeks later. The color of the acne lesions had started to fade, and they were no longer so dark red. The lesions had reduced in size and were also not as painful to the touch.

Formula Modification

Zhè bèi mǔ was reduced to 12 g, *yì yǐ rén* to 15 g, and *shí gāo* to 15 g, and *zào jiǎo cì* was increased to 9 g to move blood, in order to help the lesions fade. *Mǔ dān pí* was changed to dry-fried (*chǎo*) because this form of preparation is more suitable for the digestive system when the herb is used long-term. Because this was a case of severe acne that was difficult to treat and required more time, the patient was advised to continue drinking her herbal decoction for another three weeks. She was also told to change her eating habits by avoiding fatty and spicy food. Fast-food restaurants should be a no-go from now on! The importance of a healthy diet for improving skin problems had already been discussed with her during the first consultation; however, it seemed that this young woman didn't take that information seriously, and it had to be stressed to her again. She was reminded that the patient is always a part of the therapy. If some bad habits are not changed, Chinese herbs cannot work effectively, and this is particularly relevant for serious skin conditions.

Clinical Course

After three and a half more weeks, the patient returned to the clinic once more. She said that she was now following the dietary advice as closely as possible, although it was not always easy for her to break long-lasting habits. However, her facial skin and her hair appeared less oily, and her skin continued to improve. There were almost no inflamed pimples, no pus, and no pain. But because the active lesions on her face had been so deep, new scars were added to the old ones. This was, of course, unavoidable considering the severity of her acne. Clearing heat and draining dampness was still needed, but the focus of the prescription was slightly shifted towards moving blood to try to improve the scarring. *Yīn chén hāo* was reduced to 9 g, *qīng hāo* was removed, and *táo rén* 12 g was added. This prescription was given for another three weeks. The patient was asked to come back after four weeks to reassess her skin and adjust the formula accordingly.

#5: Female Patient, 29 Years Old–Acne
First Visit

This young female patient came into the clinic with a main complaint of facial acne, but was also experiencing premenstrual symptoms. The acne appeared on her cheeks and chin in particular as bright-red lesions, with a mix of inflamed papules and pustules. She also reported that her skin usually gets worse before her period, along with premenstrual symptoms such as mood changes, breast distension, and increased sweating with odor that lingers even after showering. She affirmed that she experiences period pain but only mildly.

The tongue showed small red dots, especially on the sides, which indicated internal heat. The tongue had tooth-marks and the tongue coating was thin and yellow. Her pulse was rapid and thready.

TCM Diagnosis

Liver Qì Stagnation Transforming into Fire (*gān yù huà huǒ* 肝郁化火).

Treatment Principle

Soothe the Liver, resolve constraint, and release heat (*shū gān jiě yù xiè rè* 疏肝解郁泄热).

Formula

Modified *Dān Zhī Xiāo Yáo Sǎn* (Moutan and Gardenia Rambling Powder):

chái hú	Bupleuri, Radix	9 g
dāng guī	Angelicae Sinensis, Radix	9 g
bái sháo	Paeonia Albiflora, Radix	9 g
bái zhú	Atractylodis Macrocephalae, Rhizoma	9 g
fú líng	Poriae Cocos, Sclerotium	9 g
zhì gān cǎo	Glycyrrhizae Preparata, Radix	4.5 g
mǔ dān pí	Moutan, Cortex	9 g
(*chǎo*) *zhī zǐ*	Gardeniae, Fructus	12 g
shēng dì huáng	Rehmanniae Glutinosae, Radix	12 g
xiāng fù	Cyperi, Rhizoma	9 g
lián qiáo	Forsythiae, Fructus	9 g

Raw herbs taken as a decoction, twice daily for 15 days.

Case Analysis

This case is a good example of how effectively classical formulas can work, and how prescriptions don't have to be complicated in order to work perfectly. It also demonstrates that many modifications are not always required when the principle is right. If the result is heading in the right direction, one can continue the treatment without needing to change many herbs or making it too complicated. The patient's acne that became worse premenstrually, along with the sweating shortly before her period, the red dots, especially on the sides of her tongue,[11] as well as the thin yellow tongue coating, all indicate that stagnant Liver qì has transformed into fire. Blocked Liver qì that cannot move freely and stagnates for a long time within the body produces heat, and if this continues for too long, it gradually turns into fire. The upward rising of fire, a yáng pathogen, always tends to first affect the head. With regard to acne, this means that the face is likely to be affected most. Modified *Dān Zhī Xiāo Yáo Sǎn* (Moutan and Gardenia Rambling Powder) was used in this case to spread the Liver qì, resolve constraint, and clear heat. This formula was explained in detail earlier in the section "Heat Stagnation in the Liver Meridian" in Chapter 5 and can be referred back to if needed. *Shēng dì huáng* was added to strengthen the action of cooling heat and draining fire without causing stasis. *Xiāng fù* regulates the Liver qì and releases constraint. It is frequently used to treat menstrual problems such as pain, breast distension, or irregular menstruation. *Lián qiáo* drains fire from constraint. Similar to *zhī zǐ*, it is light in weight, making it perfect to clear heat from the upper *jiāo*. The combination of *xiāng fù* and *lián qiáo* can also be used when a patient is irritated or bad tempered due to qì constraint with signs of heat. Please note that either *zhì gān cǎo* or *gān cǎo* can be used. And if a stronger approach is needed, one may consider using *Lóng Dǎn Xiè Gān Tāng* (Gentian Decoction to Drain the Liver). If the patient's constitution is strong enough, this formula is a good treatment option. Alternatively, if the original formula seems to be too weak and not effective enough, one may switch to a stronger formula in the course of the treatment.

Second Visit

The patient came back into the clinic two weeks later. The acne lesions were less inflamed. She was expecting her period very soon, and she reported that the breast distension, while still noticeable, was less troublesome. This showed that we were on the right track with her prescription, and so no modifications were made to the formula. The patient was advised to continue taking the same prescription for another two weeks, and then return to the clinic so the efficacy of the herbs could be assessed after her period.

Clinical Course

After two and a half more weeks, her condition was very promising. She reported that her period was relatively smooth and confirmed the positive effect of the herbs on her breast distension. She didn't report any major period pain and was managing the lead-up to her period without any major complaints. Her skin had started to heal and her complexion improved more and more. (*Chǎo*) *zhī zǐ* and *shēng dì huáng* were reduced to 9 g of each herb. She was advised to take this prescription until the end of her next period.

#6: Male Patient, Mid-40s–Rosacea
First Visit

This male patient presented with acne rosacea, manifesting as facial redness in the central area of his face, covering his nose and cheeks. Obvious telangiectasia[12] could not be seen but his skin appeared thickened, with many pustules on his face. His skin felt hot with a local burning, and the pustules were quite painful. His main concern was his nose, which appeared swollen, bumpy, and red, and so this was the primary focus of his treatment. Other skin characteristics included acne on his back, which was covered with inflamed red and deep painful pimples. It has to be mentioned that this man was not averse to alcohol and cigarettes, which, of course, was unfavorable for his condition but also a potential cause of it. He didn't have to mention it; you could smell it. Accompanying symptoms included thirst, stools that varied from loose to hard, and a tendency to feel full easily.

His tongue was red and slightly purplish. His pulse was rapid and slippery.

TCM Diagnosis
Heat in the Lungs and Stomach (*fèi wèi rè shèng* 肺胃热盛).

Treatment Principle
Clear heat in the Lungs and Stomach in order to clear the skin (*qīng fèi wèi rè yǐ qīng pí fū rè* 清肺胃热以清皮肤热).

Formula

shí gāo	Gypsum Fibrosum	30 g
zhī mǔ	Anemarrhenae, Rhizoma	6 g
(chǎo) huáng qín	Scutellariae, Radix (dry-fried)	9 g
mǔ dān pí	Moutan, Cortex	12 g
pí pá yè	Eriobotryae Japonicae, Folium	15 g
sāng bái pí	Mori, Cortex	15 g
huáng qí	Astragali, Radix	9 g
fú líng	Poriae Cocos, Sclerotium	12 g
chén pí	Citri Reticulatae, Pericarpium	9 g
bái biǎn dòu	Lablab Album, Semen	9 g
tǔ fú líng	Smilacis Glabrae, Rhizoma	30 g

Raw herbs taken as a decoction, twice daily for 14 days.

Case Analysis
As previously discussed, here we can see that two classic formulas are combined to achieve the main treatment goal: clear heat in the Lungs and

Stomach, namely *Pí Pá Qīng Fèi Yǐn* (Eriobotrya Decoction to Clear the Lung) represented by its main herbs *pí pá yè* and *sāng bái pí* to clear away heat from the Lungs, and *Bái Hǔ Tāng* (White Tiger Decoction) with *shí gāo* and *zhī mǔ* to clear heat and drain fire from the *yáng míng*. As this was an advanced stage of rosacea, all four herbs were given in relatively large dosages. In addition to these herbs, *huáng qín* was used to support draining fire and relieving toxicity, and *mǔ dān pí* to amplify the heat/fire-clearing effect, cool the blood, and also invigorate the blood in order to prevent stasis. All these actions are needed for this degree of inflammation of the skin. However, considering the accompanying symptoms the patient presented with, bringing his digestion into order was just as important as treating the inflammation on the skin. Thus, *huáng qí, fú líng, chén pí*, and *bái biǎn dòu* were added to strengthen the Spleen and the Stomach, transform dampness, and harmonize the middle *jiāo*.

The patient had been abusing his body for many years, eating unhealthily, smoking, and drinking to excess. Simply using herbs to remove the heat would not be enough in this case. His problems would definitely return unless the underlying cause was addressed, rather than only working superficially and just focusing on clearing away heat. It goes without saying that this patient was informed very precisely about which foods he should definitely avoid and which are good for him. Without changing his lifestyle, his skin won't get any better. I would like to emphasize once again that in the case of skin diseases in particular, nutritional advice always forms part of the consultation. At a minimum, the patient needs a list of what to avoid, so that they know which foods will make their condition worse. Again, patients need to understand that they are an essential part of the therapy.

Finally, *tǔ fú líng* was added at a dose of 30 g. It is a perfect herb for deep and painful acne on the back, due to its cooling and detoxifying effect. If you see deep, painful pimples on the back, always keep *tǔ fú líng* in mind for reducing redness, pain, and swelling.

Second Visit

The patient returned for his follow-up consultation two weeks later. The skin on his face hadn't changed much, with just a slight reduction in pustules and redness. But the good news was that the color of the acne lesions on his back had started to fade. The lesions on the back had become smaller and were less deep and painful to the touch. Moreover, the patient reported that he had struggled with changing his diet. Nutrition, alcohol, and nicotine in particular were discussed with him again in detail. It turned out that this patient was difficult to treat, and his lifestyle also meant that treatment would take longer to work. This had been clear from the start, but now it had been confirmed. Accordingly, the patient was advised to continue drinking his herbal decoction for another two and a half weeks.

Formula Modification

There were no major changes. *Mǔ dān pí* was changed to dry-fried (*chǎo*) because this form of preparation is more suitable for the digestive system when the herb is used long-term.

Clinical Course

I have chosen this case to show that TCM is an effective medicine but that the patient is an essential part of the therapy. Why am I saying this? After three weeks the patient returned to the clinic once more. He said that he still could not follow the dietary advice completely, and especially in times of stress it was very difficult for him to stop drinking alcohol in the evening. He felt he needed it to calm down. He was informed that this was a fallacy. Instead of calming and harmonizing him, he continues to add fuel to the fire internally–the fire that makes his skin even worse.

However, his facial skin gradually started to improve. The redness started to fade a bit and the pustules reduced, but it was not enough of a change considering he had been taking herbal decoctions for more than four and half weeks now. The only real positive was that the skin on his back improved. Without removing the factors creating the heat and inflammation, much further improvement cannot be expected. However, he was prescribed with herbs for another three weeks and asked to come back when the herbs had been taken to reassess. *Sāng bái pí* was reduced to 12 g, and *shēng dì huáng* 12 g was added in order to clear heat, cool blood, and nourish yīn.

Endnotes

1 Keratosis pilaris is a very common condition where small bumps appear on the skin. The bumps can be red, white, skintoned or darker than the normal skin. The skin is dry and feels rough and sometimes itchy. It is harmless and not contagious.

2 Bensky, D., Clavey, S., and Stöger, E. (2004) *Materia Medica*, 3rd edition. Seattle, WA: Eastland Press, p.177.

3 Bensky, D., Clavey, S., and Stöger, E. (2004) *Materia Medica*, 3rd edition. Seattle, WA: Eastland Press, p.165.

4 Bensky, D., Clavey, S., and Stöger, E. (2004) *Materia Medica*, 3rd edition. Seattle, WA: Eastland Press, p.381.

5 A detailed elaboration of the herb can be found in my article: Schmitz, S. (2013) "Jiao Gu Lan: The herb of immortality." *RCHM Journal (Register of Chinese Herbal Medicine) (UK) 10*, 2, 50–53.

6 *Yú xīng cǎo* can be used externally as wet compress, herbal wash, or even as a spray in many skin diseases. It is gentle but effective and can be used for skin conditions including acne, facial dermatitis, or eczema.

7 See the section "The Natural Skin Surface Potential of Hydrogen (pH)" in Chapter 1 for the explanation of the so-called Wood's lamp which uses transillumination (light) to detect bacterial or fungal skin infections. This test is also known as the black light test or the ultraviolet light (UV) test. The UV light will cause the organisms to fluoresce.

8 Bensky, D., Clavey, S., and Stöger, E. (2004) *Materia Medica*, 3rd edition. Seattle, WA: Eastland Press, p.740.

9 Bensky, D., Clavey, S., and Stöger, E. (2004) *Materia Medica*, 3rd edition. Seattle, WA: Eastland Press, p.956.

10 Also known as Bamboo Leaves and Gypsum Combination.

11 The borders of the tongue correspond with the Liver in Chinese medicine.

12 A chronic dilation of blood vessels, also called spider veins.

Afterword

I HAVE SHARED with you my knowledge from my many years of experience in dermatology and the treatment of acne. I am sure you will see you can treat it, too. It's not difficult and it's not magic. However, it does require constant training and the will for self-improvement when things don't go well. Be flexible and keep it simple! TCM offers us an outstanding medicine for the treatment of many skin diseases. As TCM practitioners, we can be proud of this outstanding system of knowledge that we can apply in practice. Adopt this point of view confidently when talking to your patients and they will trust you. Good luck to you all!

Sabine Schmitz
December 2020

Appendix I: The External Treatment of Acne with Chinese Herbal Medicine

THIS APPENDIX provides a brief outline of external treatment options for both acne vulgaris and acne rosacea, and describes in detail how to prepare them. This is useful for practitioners who are able to make them but also for TCM pharmacists. It can also serve as useful background information you can share with your patients.

At this point it is important to mention that all suggestions given in this appendix serve as a practical guide. Don't stick to the exact prescriptions–be flexible! Different formulas can be used for various TCM patterns. The dosages and combinations can be adjusted; and multiple forms of treatment can be applied in the same session–for example, a wash first and a facial mask afterwards.

Individual Tailored Herbal Washes or Wet Compresses[1]

Washes or compresses are usually the best treatment option for both acne and rosacea. I don't recommend the use of creams as they can clog the pores and create a favorable environment for the growth of bacteria, something we want to prevent in any case!

In general, if you create your own herbal prescription for a wash or a wet compress, no more than three or four herbs are needed. Herbs can be changed as required, dosages can be adjusted–be flexible. Likewise, the volume of water used in the boiling process can be adjusted in order to vary the concentration of the medicinal liquid. Always increase the amount of water in proportion to the quantity of herbs. This applies to all the external applications described in this book. Use 10–15 g of each herb you have selected, keeping in mind that a maximum of 100 ml of water is used per 10 g of herbs. If you are using three herbs, for example, a maximum of

300 ml of water would be used. Soak the herbs in water for 15–20 minutes. Bring them to a boil, and then reduce the heat, allowing the herbs to simmer slowly for approximately 15–20 minutes. Strain the liquid and store it in the fridge. Wash the face with the liquid twice a day, or, ideally, apply it as a wet (cold) compress on the affected skin lesions for 15 minutes, once or twice (sometimes even three times) a day. Please advise your patient to use each compress just once, a make-up removal pad is suitable for this, and to not contaminate the fresh liquid with already used materials. The best way is to pour a little of the decoction into a small bowl each time and dip the compress into this. Once the treatment has been completed, discard the excess liquid. This prevents any bacterial contamination from unclean application.

Some additional advice for boiling times for external applications: Do not boil herbs used for external therapy longer than 30 minutes. As the ingredients are intended to work on the surface, only a light cooking process is required. The standard practice is a boiling time of approximately 15–20 minutes. Decoctions taken internally generally have to work at a deeper level in the body and therefore they require a longer boiling process in order to reach their required depth.

With regard to the temperature, use lukewarm or cold water for a wash or compress, never warm or even hot water. Imagine how painful the patients' skin is. The skin often feels very hot with a burning sensation. The effect of an external application in the treatment of acne or rosacea should always be to calm the skin, and ideally to eliminate the inflammation. Only cool liquid can do this. Hot water would definitely make the condition worse instead of giving the patient relief. This is very important!

Some notes on specific herbs for external application:

Zhāng Nǎo

One example for a simple herbal compress, which is very often prescribed for acne relief, is a wash consisting only of *zhāng nǎo* (camphor). It seems to get very good results in relieving pain, swelling, and irritation in deep and painful pimples. It has to be used with caution, however, because *zhāng nǎo* is suitable for external applications only. Patients should be informed that it is toxic if taken internally! It should be also used with care for people with skin allergies.

For application, grind *zhāng nǎo* into a fine powder and mix it thoroughly with warm water to dissolve (do not decoct). Apply a wet (cold) compress once or twice a day for about 15 minutes each time on the affected skin lesions. If the skin feels tight or dry afterwards, discontinue use of this herb. According to my clinical experience, patients can react very differently to *zhāng nǎo*.

Liú Huáng

Another example of an herbal wash or wet compress is *liú huáng* (sulphur). Sulphur clears heat, reduces toxicity, invigorates blood, and stops itching. As it can relieve inflammation, it is often given in cases of bacterial super-infection. While I have seen this used in China, I have not often used sulphur as an herbal wash or wet compress in my practice. However, I wanted to share this information with you, so that you can test it for yourself if needed.

Aloe Vera

Aloe vera is a very useful home remedy. It has already been discussed in Chapter 8. I often recommend it to patients with rosacea as an additional treatment, either after an external herbal wash or compress, or before using their normal skincare products. Aloe vera has a cooling effect, soothing the skin and relieving redness and itching due to inflammation. It supports skin regeneration and has a moisturizing effect. It is mainly used as a gel, taken straight out of the refrigerator. Patients with rosacea often report that using cool aloe vera gives them immediate relief. In ordinary acne, however, aloe vera is rarely recommended.

Shí Gāo

Shí gāo can be used as a wet compress or a facial mask. It is most suitable for patients with serious acne rosacea, but can be also applied in cases of acne when the face is very red and the skin feels hot and inflamed. Facial masks are usually prepared with honey as a standard base. With *shí gāo*, however, it is possible to work in many different ways. You can use honey as a base, but the powder can also be mixed with green tea. If neither honey nor green tea is available, use boiled water to prepare a thin paste and store it in an airtight container. Apply the paste once or twice a day on the affected areas as a facial mask. It clears heat and drains fire, and it feels very cooling on the skin, providing immediate relief.

Please note that, like *shí gāo*, any other herbal combination can be prepared as a facial mask. If you work with powdered herbs, the best standard bases for facial masks are honey, green tea, or water. If you work with decoctions, standard bases can be pearl powder, made from powdered *zhēn zhū mǔ*, or, quite simply healing earth (healing clay). Some sources mention that pastes should be gently rubbed over the skin on the face. If a patient has a serious skin condition such as acne or rosacea, I would refrain from rubbing in order to avoid injuring the skin. Thus, it is recommended to gently apply the paste and leave it on the skin for about 15–30 minutes. The duration of application can be shorter or longer, and can vary depending on patients' needs.

Popular Formulas for External Treatments

For clarity, the formulas will be listed alphabetically. Moreover, different forms of application will be described for each formula to give you the largest possible selection from which you can then choose the form that is most suitable for your patients.

Cuó Chuāng Xǐ Jì (Acne (Wash) Lotion)

liú huáng	Sulphur	6 g
zhāng nǎo	Camphora	10 g
xī huáng shī jiāo	Astragalus, Gummifer	1 g
	Lime Water	1 liter

This formula has been mentioned in the *Zhōng Yī Wài Kē Xué* (Traditional Chinese Medicine Surgery), written by Zhū Rén-Kāng.[2] *Xī huáng shī jiāo* (gum tragacanth) mainly serves as a viscosity regulator but is not available everywhere. In Germany, for example, it is not available. Thus, I suggest using this combination with all other ingredients but omitting the gum. In this case, I would call it a "wash" instead of a "lotion," due to its changed consistency without the gum. The efficacy, however, remains the same.

For application, grind the ingredients to a fine powder and mix them thoroughly with the lime water. Gently apply the lotion to the affected areas of the skin after cleansing the face in the evening. It clears heat, reduces toxicity, invigorates blood, stops pain, and eases itching. As it can relieve inflammation, this combination can be given in case of bacterial super-infection.

This lotion is very effective but it should be used with care. Patients must be informed about the color and the smell of *liú huáng*, in order to warn them of these downsides before usage.[3] And again, *zhāng nǎo* is toxic if taken internally!

Diān Dǎo Sǎn (Upside Down Powder) and *Diān Dǎo Sǎn Xǐ Jì* (Upside Down Powder Wash Lotion)

| *dà huáng* | Rhei, Radix et Rhizoma | 10 g |
| *liú huáng* | Sulphur | 10 g |

Grind equal quantities of the herbs into a fine powder and mix them thoroughly. This is called *Diān Dǎo Sǎn* (Upside Down Powder). For application, mix the powder with 150–200 ml of cool boiled water or green tea into a thin paste. If the lesions are smaller, use lower dosages of herbs and less liquid, and vice versa. Gently apply a thin layer of the paste on the affected areas of the skin with clean fingertips or a sterile cotton ball after cleansing the face in the evening, and wash it off the next morning with clean water. *Diān Dǎo Sǎn* disperses inflammation, clears heat, reduces fire, cools and invigorates the blood, purges toxins, and stops itching. It can be used as a basic treatment of acne for all TCM patterns, and other combinations or formulas can be used at the same time if this is not enough. Be careful in the treatment of sensitive patients because of *liú huáng*'s color and smell. Irritation is relatively rare, but if there is an allergic reaction, immediately stop this application. When working with very sensitive patients, it is best to start gently and then gradually extend the application time.

If mixed with lime water[4] (usually about 1 liter), the combination is then called *Diān Dǎo Sǎn Xǐ Jì* (Upside Down Powder Wash Lotion). This is probably the most common form of application of *Diān Dǎo Sǎn* in the treatment of acne. Apply *Diān Dǎo Sǎn Xǐ Jì* at least once or twice a day on the affected areas of the skin; rinse off but avoid using soap as it tends to clog the pores. This combination clears heat and cools the blood. It can be used as a wet compress as well. Apply the liquid by using a compress (gauze pad) or cloth and leave it to dry on the skin for about 20 minutes, once or twice a day.

Hēi Bù Yào Gāo (Black Cloth Medicated Paste)[5]

lǎo hēi cù	Atrum Vetum, Acetum	2500 ml
wǔ bèi zǐ	Rhois Chinensis, Galla	840 g
wú gōng	Scolopendra	10 pieces
bīng piàn	Borneolum	3 g
fēng mì	Mel	180 g

This formula was invented by Professor Zhào Bǐng-Nán.[6] Prof. Zhào worked extensively on creating new treatment options for many patients with various skin conditions, including acne. The work of Prof. Zhào has greatly benefited Chinese dermatology. Although some of the ingredients may be restricted or forbidden in some countries, I am mentioning this formula because of its effectiveness in improving the appearance of skin prone to the formation of keloid scars. It helps to smooth the skin while improving the skin's appearance and is best used for acne due to phlegm and blood stasis.

For application, grind each herb separately to a fine powder. Then boil the black vinegar for about 30 minutes, add the honey to the vinegar and boil again for about one minute. After that, gradually add the fine herbal powder of *wǔ bèi zǐ* and let it cook over gentle heat. Stir constantly always in the same direction until the texture is thick. Now, add *wú gōng* and *bīng piàn*. The result should be a black, shiny, and soft paste. Pour the paste into a glass or porcelain container. No metal container should be used. Apply a small amount over the affected areas of the skin and allow to dry fully once or twice a day. A black film will form, which should gently be washed off with warm water.

Hóng Huā Gāo (Safflower Ointment)

hóng huā	Carthami, Flos	2 g
dān shēn	Salviae Miltiorhizae, Radix	2 g
chuān xiōng	Chuanxiong, Rhizoma	2 g
zhāng nǎo	Camphora	2 g

These quantities will produce an ointment of 100 ml. In making your own ointments, it is important to know exactly what ingredients are being used. Only pure, natural, environmentally friendly options should be selected, ensuring that the ingredients do not irritate the skin and are suitable for sensitive skincare. Furthermore, if there is an ingredient a patient is allergic to, it can simply be left out or replaced with something else. Some practitioners may like to use petroleum jelly for making this ointment. In this case, 93 g of petroleum jelly should be used. In Chinese dermatology, however, it is recommended to refrain from using petroleum jelly, even though it is still often mentioned in medical textbooks. As previously mentioned, petroleum jelly is not a high-quality solution. There are many alternatives that are higher in quality, natural, light in texture, more easily spread, and more pleasant on the skin, such as jojoba oil, sesame oil (*zhī má yóu*), or native olive oil.

For application, grind the ingredients to a fine powder and soak them in 100 ml of sesame oil (or any other high-quality oil) for at least 24 hours. Bring to a boil over gentle heat in order for the ingredients to dissolve, then allow to cool. Filter off the herb-infused sesame oil, leave it to set, and apply the ointment once or twice a day on the affected areas of the skin. I have given you the instructions with 100 ml of oil instead of making it overly complicated with the use of the original 93 ml of oil. All proportions can be changed as needed anyway. If a thicker consistency is required, just melt a very small amount of beeswax into the prepared ointment.

In general, all ointments can also be prepared as creams. For creams, the sesame oil is replaced with natural thickeners of beeswax, cocoa butter, or shea butter, which gives them a more solid texture. The proportions can be varied according to individual needs; there are no strict specifications regarding ratios. In acne, however, I prefer to work with lighter textures when making medical external applications. In cosmetics, it is different. For cosmetics, a thicker texture is more appropriate for day and night creams. It is also important to mention at this point that there is a big increase in effectiveness when the herbs are ground (pulverized). The process of grinding enlarges the surface area, enabling much more substance to enter the decoction during the soaking and cooking process. In practice, we have found that oil-based lotions that have not been ground or pulverized are not as powerful and effective.

Huà Dú Săn Gāo (Toxicity Transforming Powder Paste)

huáng lián	Coptidis, Rhizoma	60 g
rŭ xiāng	Olibanum, Gummi	60 g
mò yào	Myrrha	60 g
chuān bèi mŭ	Fritillariae Cirrhosae, Bulbus	60 g

tiān huā fěn	Trichosanthis, Radix	120 g
dà huáng	Rhei, Radix et Rhizoma	120 g
chì sháo	Paeoniae Rubrae, Radix	120 g
xióng huáng	Realgar	60 g
gān cǎo	Glycyrrhizae Uralensis, Radix	45 g
niú huáng	Bovis Calculus	12 g
bīng piàn	Borneolum	15 g

This formula is called *Huà Dú Sǎn* (Toxicity Transforming Powder). Two substances in the formula are not available outside of China, namely *xióng huáng* and *niú huáng*. *Xióng huáng* might be replaced with *liú huáng* as both substances can resolve toxicity. The prescription can, however, be used without *xióng huáng* and *niú huáng*, and would still be strong enough to clear heat, remove toxins, promote blood circulation, and resolve swelling. It is quite often used in acne that shows serious inflammation, nodules, and cysts.

Both formulas, *Huà Dú Sǎn* and *Huà Dú Sǎn Gāo*, originate from Professor Zhào Bǐng-Nán. He recorded these formulas in the *Zhào Bǐng-Nán Lín Chuáng Jīng Yàn Jí* (Zhào Bǐng-Nán's Clinical Experience Set).[7] While the original prescription recommends petroleum jelly as a carrier, the use of natural substances is always preferable. As already mentioned, petroleum jelly is not a high-quality solution. Let me describe how to make *Huà Dú Sǎn Gāo* without the use of petroleum jelly. For application, grind the ingredients of *Huà Dú Sǎn* to a fine powder and mix them thoroughly. To make *Huà Dú Sǎn Gāo*, about 50 g of the powder should be sufficient for use on the face. Mix it well with 150 ml of sesame oil or any other organic base. Apply the paste once or twice a day on the affected areas of the skin. Please don't forget that all pastes can be prepared with oil or with water. When preparing a paste with water, just use boiled water instead of sesame oil. As simple as that! Although it is not advised in classic books, I am sure that high-quality green tea as a base would also work.

As an alternative to a paste, one may prepare it as an oil-based ointment. Grind the ingredients of *Huà Dú Sǎn* to a fine powder and mix them thoroughly. Soak the herbs in a proportion of 1:4 in sesame oil for about 24 hours. The next day, bring it to a boil over gentle heat, filter off the herb-infused sesame oil, and allow to gel. Before applying on the skin, it can be mixed with a small amount of beeswax to make a thicker ointment, but this is not essential. Apply the ointment once or twice a day on the affected areas of the skin. Because TCM is so flexible, this combination can also be used as a wash. Simply boil the herbs in water for a maximum of 20 minutes, strain, and use as a wash.

Huáng Qín Gāo (Scutellariae Baicalensis Paste)

huáng qín	Scutellariae, Radix	10 g
dà huáng	Rhei, Radix et Rhizoma	10 g
huáng bǎi	Phellodendri, Cortex	10 g
kǔ shēn	Sophorae Flavescentis, Radix	10 g

All ingredients are used in equal parts. The quantities mentioned above serve as an example, and can be increased or decreased depending on the size of the skin areas needing to be treated. Grind the ingredients to a fine powder and mix them thoroughly with sesame oil or any other organic base into a paste. Apply the paste once or twice a day on the affected areas of the skin. Leave it on for about 15–30 minutes and then gently wash it off afterwards. Always keep in mind that all given timelines can be varied–shortened or lengthened; the paste can even be left on overnight. You decide what is needed according to the treatment case.

Huáng Qín Gāo is best used in acne cases with obvious pus, when the lesions are red, swollen, and feel hot and painful. It clears heat, dries dampness, reduces swelling, and stops itching. When the inflammation is reduced, the skin can heal faster.

Jiě Dú Xǐ Gāo (Detoxifying Lotion)[8]

pú gōng yīng	Taraxaci, Herba	30 g
kǔ shēn	Sophorae Flavescentis, Radix	12 g
huáng bǎi	Phellodendri, Cortex	12 g
lián qiáo	Forsythiae, Fructus	12 g
mù biē zǐ[9]	Momordicae, Semen	12 g
jīn yín huā	Lonicerae Japonicae, Flos	10 g
bái zhǐ	Angelica Dahuricae, Radix	10 g
chì sháo	Paeoniae Rubrae, Radix	10 g
mǔ dān pí	Moutan, Cortex	10 g
gān cǎo	Glycyrrhizae Uralensis, Radix	10 g

Please note that some sources[10] mention this formula with *mù biē zǐ*, some with *ér chá* (Catechu) instead, and some may even mention it without any of these substances. As both substances are not available in every country, it is absolutely fine and still very effective when prepared without these two herbs.

To prepare a wash or a wet compress, soak the ingredients in 1.5 liters of water for 20 minutes. Bring them to a boil, and then reduce to a low heat, allowing the herbs to simmer slowly for approximately 20 minutes, and then strain the liquid. For application, wash the affected area or apply a wet compress on the affected skin lesions two to three times a day for about 15 minutes each time, adjusting the time as needed. To prepare an oil-based paste, grind the ingredients to a fine powder and mix it thoroughly with sesame oil. Green tea can be used as an alternative to oil, as can boiled water. This herbal combination strongly clears heat, resolves toxicity, invigorates the blood, and reduces swelling. It is quite effective in any form of acne that is accompanied with severe inflammation, pus, and risk of scarring.

Jīn Huáng Sǎn (Golden Yellow Powder)[11]

dà huáng	Rhei, Radix et Rhizoma	10 g
huáng bǎi	Phellodendri, Cortex	10 g
jiāng huáng	Curcumae Longae, Rhizoma	10 g
bái zhǐ	Angelica Dahuricae, Radix	5–10 g
tiān nán xīng	Arisaematis, Rhizoma	5–10 g
chén pí	Citri Reticulatae, Pericarpium	5–10 g
cāng zhú	Atractylodis, Rhizoma	5–10 g
hòu pò	Magnoliae Officinalis, Cortex	5–10 g
gān cǎo	Glycyrrhizae Uralensis, Radix	5–10 g
tiān huā fěn	Trichosanthis, Radix	10–15 g

This combination is called *Jīn Huáng Sǎn* (Golden Yellow Powder). The quantities mentioned above serve as an example. Vary the quantities and proportions in order to alter the effect, and increase the amounts if larger skin areas need to be treated. For application, grind the ingredients to a fine powder and mix it thoroughly with sesame oil or any other organic base such as honey, tea (green tea is best), or even boiled chrysanthemum (*jú huā*) water. Then cover the affected area with the resulting paste. As you can see, the options for making a paste from the powder are very diverse.

This combination can be also used as a wet compress after decocting the ingredients for 20 minutes in water and filtering the herbs off. Don't stick to the doses listed above; instead, try variations in order to get the best effect.

Jīn Huáng Sǎn is a very effective formula when toxic heat is involved. It clears heat, removes toxins, dispels dampness, eliminates blood stasis, and reduces swelling. It is thus very useful for acne with red and hot swollen lesions, and inflamed painful skin with sensations of burning and itching. Typically, the acne lesions have not yet come to a head and are very deep and painful. We have all seen this in our patients.

Jiǔ Zhā Bí Gāo (Rosacea Paste)[12]

mì tuó sēng	Lithargyrum	60 g
xuán shēn	Scrophulariae Ningpoensis, Radix	30 g
liú huáng	Sulphur	30 g
qīng fěn	Calomelas	24 g

Mì tuó sēng is toxic and is therefore regarded as an obsolete ingredient in most countries outside China. When working topically, *mì tuó sēng* can be replaced with *qiān dān* (Minium, where this is available).[13] Otherwise, prepare the paste with the other three ingredients.

For application, grind the ingredients to a fine powder and mix with honey to form a paste. Store in an airtight jar. Clean the face and gently rub with the paste for five minutes in the morning and again before bedtime. This combination can be also used as a wet compress. If using it as a wet compress, reduce the dosages accordingly. The application time would then be 15–30 minutes depending how sensitive the patient is. Remember to work carefully with substances such as *liú huáng*. *Jiǔ Zhā Bí Gāo* absorbs fluids (pus), reduces swelling, and eliminates toxins. It is often used for severe cases of rosacea with red and hot-feeling skin, papules, pustules, and rhinophyma. In addition, it also kills parasites.[14]

Pí Shī Yī Gāo (Pus Absorbing Ointment)

(*duàn*) *shí gāo*	(calcinated) Gypsum Fibrosum	20 g
dì yú	Sanguisorbae, Radix	10 g
bái fán	Alumen	10 g

This formula comes from the book *Zhū Rén Kāng Lín Chuáng Jīng Yàn Jí* (A Collection of Zhu Rén-Kāng's Clinical Experiences, 1979), written by Zhū Rén-Kāng.[15] As the name of the formula states, its function is clearing heat, absorbing discharge (pus), and relieving itching. It is suitable for any form of acne in which red, thick, edematous, inflamed, and very painful lesions in the form of papules, papulopustules, and/or pustules are seen. Dr Zhū suggested preparing the powder with petroleum jelly. However, when a discharge-absorbing action is needed, I would always suggest preparing a formula as a wash, wet compress, or ointment. A thick and hardly spreadable cream would be not advisable as the discharge has to be drained, not occluded. A thick substance like petroleum jelly would prevent this and keep inside what should be discharged. An inflammatory process could certainly worsen as a result.

To prepare this formula as an ointment, grind all substances to a fine powder. Mix them thoroughly with a liquid such as sesame oil, and apply two or three times a day on the affected skin lesions. Alternatively, dissolve the substances in water for a topical wash. You might also use this formula as a wet compress, gently applied on the affected skin areas. Please note that mineral substances such as *bái fán* can be ground to a fine powder for direct use on the skin.

Sān Huáng Xǐ Jì (Three Yellow Cleanser Formula)

dà huáng	Rhei, Radix et Rhizoma	10 g
huáng bǎi	Phellodendri, Cortex	10 g
huáng qín	Scutellariae, Radix	10 g
kǔ shēn	Sophorae Flavescentis, Radix	10 g

There are two ways in which to prepare this formula.

First method: Soak the ingredients in 500 ml of water for 20–30 minutes. Bring them to a boil, and then reduce to a low heat, allowing the herbs to simmer slowly for approximately 20 minutes, then strain the liquid. For application, wash the affected area or apply as a wet compress two or three times a day, for 15–20 minutes each time. *Sān Huáng Xǐ Jì* can be also applied with a sterile cotton ball, up to three or four times a day. It clears heat, relieves inflammation, arrests secretion, and stops itching. In clinic, this manifests as acne with papules and pustules with red, hot, and burning skin lesions, sometimes accompanied by pain and/or itching. If there are erupted acne lesions, add *pú gōng yīng*, depending on the individual needs of your patient.

Second method: Grind the ingredients to a fine powder. Take 10–15 g of the powder and suspend in 100 ml of distilled water and 1 ml of phenol. Shake the preparation well before use and apply to the lesions. As this method seems too complicated and I'm not fond of chemicals, I definitely prefer the first preparation method.

Sì Huáng Gāo (Four Yellow Paste)

huáng qín	Scutellariae, Radix	30 g
huáng lián	Coptidis, Rhizoma	30 g
huáng bǎi	Phellodendri, Cortex	10 g
dà huáng	Rhei, Radix et Rhizoma	30 g
zé lán	Lycopi, Herba	30 g
huáng là	Yellow Wax (Beeswax)	125g
zhī má yóu	Sesame Oil	250 ml

This formula also originated from the book *Zhū Rén Kāng Lín Chuáng Jīng Yàn Jí* (A Collection of Zhu Rén-Kāng's Clinical Experiences, 1979), written by Zhū Rén-Kāng. The name "*Sì Huáng*" is given because the first four of the Chinese names of its ingredients contain the word *huáng*, which means yellow. *Sì* is the Chinese word for the number four. All these herbs are bitter and cold in flavor and nature. They clear heat and drain fire. *Sì Huáng Gāo* can be effectively used for the treatment of hot toxic skin lesions, in particular acne lesions that show severe inflammation, are purulent, and tend to form scars. Due to the presence of *zé lán*, it can also be used when nodules and cysts are involved. This is because the herb invigorates the blood and dispels stasis, and can therefore relieve painful skin lesions and swelling.

For application, melt the yellow wax and the sesame oil over moderate heat. Grind all other ingredients to a fine powder and stir into the oil (after removing the pot from the heat) to form a paste. Allow to cool and gently apply the paste once or twice a day to the affected areas of the skin. The paste should be left on for about 20–30 minutes, then gently wash it off with clean water. Always work gently as the patient's skin tends to be very sensitive and inflamed, and usually feels very painful.

Zào Shī Xǐ Gāo (Damp-Heat Eliminating Ointment)

bái xiān pí	Dictamni Radicis, Cortex	10g
mǎ chǐ xiàn	Portulacae, Herba	10 g
kǔ shēn	Sophorae Flavescentis, Radix	10 g
huáng bǎi	Phellodendri, Cortex	10 g
cāng zhú	Atractylodis, Rhizoma	10 g

For application, grind the ingredients to a fine powder. Soak them in 300 ml of sesame oil for two or three days, then cook over gentle heat for a short time. Filter off the herbal residues and allow the oil to cool before applying to the skin. Apply the ointment two or three times a day to the affected areas of the skin. Please note that the ointment can be mixed with beeswax to get a thicker consistency before applying to the skin. It can also be prepared as a wash or a wet compress. For that, soak the ingredients in about 500 ml of water for 20 minutes. Bring them to a boil, and then reduce to a low flame allowing the herbs to simmer slowly for approximately 20 minutes and at the end, strain the liquid. For application, wash the affected area or apply a wet compress to the affected skin lesions two to three times a day for about 15 minutes each time.

This formula clears heat and thus relieves irritation, dispels wind and thus eases itching, and dries dampness and thus improves swelling. It is frequently used not just for acne but also for eczema, urticaria, etc.

Zǐ Yún Gāo (Purple Cloud Ointment)[16]

| *zǐ cǎo* | Arnebiae Seu Lithospermi, Radix | 15 g |
| *dāng guī* | Angelicae Sinensis, Radix | 10–15 g |

Grind *dāng guī* to a fine powder, add *zǐ cǎo*, and mix it well with 100–150 ml of sesame oil. Soak for three or four days. The herbs then become soft and only have to be boiled for a very short time over gentle heat. Remove the herbal residues as usual and allow the oil to cool. It can be mixed with beeswax or creams before applying to the skin. Apply the ointment once or twice a day to the affected areas of the skin. This formula can also be used as a wash. It helps skin healing and speeds up the excretion of toxins. Sometimes *gān cǎo* is added to the formula. *Gān cǎo* harmonizes the other herbs and is very good at reducing toxicity.

Endnotes

1 All suggestions for external use are a starting point and can be adjusted according to your own preferences and, of course, to the patient's individual needs.

2 *Zhōng Yī Wài Kē Xué* (Traditional Chinese Medicine Surgery), written by Zhū Rén-Kāng. Beijing: People's Medical Publishing House, 1987.

3 Prescribe with caution for internal use. If used internally, use very low dosages and in prepared form. Otherwise, sulphur is toxic in high oral doses (10–20 g). Source: Bensky, D., Clavey, S., and Stöger, E. (2004) *Materia Medica*, 3rd edition. Seattle, WA: Eastland Press, p.1025.

4 If no lime water is available, cold boiled water or green tea will do!

5 May contain herbs that are restricted or forbidden in some countries.

6 Professor Zhào Bǐng-Nán (Chinese: 赵炳南, 1899–1984).

7 *Zhào Bǐng-Nán Lín Chuáng Jīng Yàn Jí* (Zhào Bǐng-Nán's Clinical Experience Set). Beijing: People's Medical Publishing House, 1975.

8 If available.

9 If available.

10 The sources here vary but it seems that the original formula comes from the Shandong University of Traditional Chinese Medicine, Jinan, China.

11 External application only, usually used as a paste or plaster.

12 The formula is named according to its action: A paste (*gāo*) that treats rosacea (*jiǔ zhā bí*). The combination is mentioned in: Bensky, D., Clavey, S., and Stöger, E. (2004) *Materia Medica*, 3rd edition. Seattle, WA: Eastland Press, p.1062.

13 Bensky, D., Clavey, S., and Stöger, E. (2004) *Materia Medica*, 3rd edition. Seattle, WA: Eastland Press, p.1062.

14 *Mi tuó sēng* and *qīng fěn*.

15 *Zhū Rén Kāng Lín Chuáng Jīng Yàn Jí* (A Collection of Zhu Rén-Kāng's Clinical Experiences), written by Zhū Rén-Kāng. Beijing: People's Medical Publishing House, 1979.

16 May contain herbs that are restricted or forbidden in some countries. Unfortunately, *zǐ cǎo* (Arnebiae Seu Lithospermi, Radix) is not available in Germany.

Appendix II: *Pīnyīn*–Chinese–English Formula Cross-Reference

Pīnyīn	Chinese	English
Bái Hǔ Tāng	白虎汤	White Tiger Decoction
Bái Liǎn Gāo Tú Fāng	白蔹膏涂方	Ampelopsis Root Cream
Chái Hú Shū Gān Sǎn	柴胡疏肝散	Bupleurum Powder to Spread the Liver
Cuó Chuāng Jiān Jì	痤疮煎剂	Acne Decoction
Cuó Chuāng Xǐ Jì	痤疮洗剂	Acne (Wash) Lotion
Dān Zhī Xiāo Yáo Sǎn	丹栀逍遥散	Moutan and Gardenia Rambling Powder
Diān Dǎo Sǎn	颠倒散	Upside Down Powder
Diān Dǎo Sǎn Xǐ Jì	颠倒散洗剂	Upside Down Powder Wash Lotion
Dōng Kuí Sǎn	冬葵散	Cluster Mallow Fruit Powder
Èr Chén Tāng	二陈汤	Decoction of Two Old (Cured) Drugs
Fáng Fēng Tōng Shèng Sǎn	防风通圣散	Ledebouriella Sage-Inspired Powder
Gǎo Běn Sǎn	藁本散	Ligustici Sinensis Powder
Hǎi Zǎo Yù Hú Tāng	海藻玉壶汤	Sargassum Decoction for the Jade Flask
Hēi Bù Yào Gāo	黑布药膏	Black Cloth Medicated Paste
Hóng Huā Gāo	红花膏	Safflower Ointment
Huà Dú Sǎn	化毒散	Toxicity Transforming Powder
Huà Dú Sǎn Gāo	化毒散膏	Toxicity Transforming Powder Paste
Huáng Lián Jiě Dú Tāng	黄连解毒汤	Coptis Decoction to Relieve Toxicity

Pīnyīn	Chinese	English
Huáng Qín Gāo	黄芩膏	Scutellariae Baicalensis Paste
Jiā Wèi Xiāo Yáo Sǎn	加味逍遥散	Moutan and Gardenia Rambling Powder
Jiāng Cán Sǎn	僵蚕散	Silkworm Powder
Jiě Dú Xǐ Gāo	解毒洗膏	Detoxifying Lotion
Jīn Huáng Sǎn	金黄散	Golden Yellow Powder
Jiǔ Zhā Bí Gāo	酒渣鼻膏	Rosacea Paste
Liáng Xuè Sì Wù Tāng	凉血四物汤	Cool the Blood with Four Substances Decoction
Liáng Xuè Wǔ Huā Tāng	凉血五花汤	Cool the Blood Decoction with Five Flowers
Liù Wèi Dì Huáng Wán	六味地黄丸	Six Ingredient Pill with Rehmannia
Mù Lán Gāo Fāng	木兰膏方	Blond Magnolia Cream (Mu Lan Cream)
Pào Chuāng Fāng	疱疮方	Blister and Sore Formula
Pí Pá Qīng Fèi Yǐn	枇杷清肺饮	Eriobotrya Decoction to Clear the Lung
Pí Shī Yī Gāo	皮湿一膏	Pus Absorbing Ointment
Qīng Fèi Sǎn	清肺散	Clear the Lungs Powder
Sān Huáng Xǐ Jì	三黄洗剂	Three Yellow Cleanser Formula
Shēn Líng Bái Zhú Sǎn	参苓白朮散	Ginseng, Poria, and Atractylodis Macrocephalae Powder
Shēng Má Bái Zhǐ Tāng	升麻白芷汤	Rhizoma Cimicifugae and Radix Angelicae Dahuricae Decoction
Sì Huáng Gāo	四黄膏	Four Yellow Paste
Sì Wù Tāng	四物汤	Four Substance Decoction
Táo Hóng Sì Wù Tāng	桃红四物汤	Four Substance Decoction with Safflower and Peach Kernel
Tōng Qiào Huó Xuè Tāng	通窍活血汤	Unblock the Orifices and Invigorate the Blood Decoction
Wǔ Bèi Zǐ Gāo	五倍子膏	Nutgall Paste
Wǔ Wèi Xiāo Dú Yǐn	五味消毒饮	Five Ingredient Decoction to Eliminate Toxins
Xiāo Yáo Sǎn	逍遥散	Rambling Powder
Xuān Cǎo Gāo Tú Fāng	萱草膏涂方	Day Lily Cream
Xuè Fǔ Zhú Yū Tāng	血府逐瘀汤	Drive Out Stasis in the Mansion of Blood Decoction
Yīn Chén Hāo Tāng	茵陈蒿汤	Artemisiae Scopariae Decoction
Yù Jī Sǎn	玉肌散	Jade Skin Powder

Pīnyīn	Chinese	English
Zào Shī Xǐ Gāo	燥湿洗膏	Damp-Heat Eliminating Ointment
Zhì Fěn Cì Jí Miàn Chuāng Fāng	治粉刺及面疮方	Acne and Facial Sore Formula
Zhì Miàn Pào Fāng	治面疱方	Facial Acne Treatment
Zhì Miàn Shàng Pào Zǐ Fāng	治面上疱子方	Facial Blister Formula
Zhì Miàn Zhā Fāng	治面渣方	Treating Facial Sore
Zhú Yè Shí Gāo Tāng	竹叶石膏汤	Lophatherus and Gypsum Decoction
Zǐ Yún Gāo	紫云膏	Purple Cloud Ointment

Appendix III: *Pīnyīn*–Chinese–Pharmaceutical Herb Cross-Reference

Pīnyīn	Chinese	Pharmaceutical
bái biǎn dòu	白扁豆	Lablab Album, Semen
bái fán	白矾	Alumen
bái fù zǐ	白附子	Typhonii, Rhizoma
bái huā shé shé cǎo	百花蛇舌草	Hedyotis Diffusae, Herba
bái liǎn	白蔹	Ampelopsis, Radix
bái sháo	白芍	Paeonia Albiflora, Radix
bái shí zhī	白石脂	Kaolinitum
bái xiān pí	白鲜皮	Dictamni Radicis, Cortex
bái zhǐ	白芷	Angelica Dahuricae, Radix
bái zhú	白术	Atractylodis Macrocephalae, Rhizoma
bǎi zǐ rén	柏子仁	Platycladi, Semen
bàn xià	半夏	Pinelliae, Rhizoma
bīng piàn	冰片	Borneolum
bò hé	薄荷	Menthae, Herba
cāng zhú	苍术	Atractylodis, Rhizoma
chái hú	柴胡	Bupleuri, Radix
chē qián cǎo	车前草	Plantaginis, Herba
chē qián zǐ	车前子	Plantaginis, Semen
chén pí	陈皮	Citri Reticulatae, Pericarpium
chì sháo	赤芍	Paeoniae Rubrae, Radix
chì xiǎo dòu	赤小豆	Phaseoli, Semen
chóng lóu	重楼	Paridis, Rhizoma
chuān bèi mǔ	川贝母	Fritillariae Cirrhosae, Bulbus

Pīnyīn	Chinese	Pharmaceutical
chuān xiōng	川芎	Chuanxiong, Rhizoma
cōng bái	葱白	Allii Fistulosi, Bulbus
dà fù pí	大腹皮	Arecae, Pericarpium
dà huáng	大黄	Rhei, Radix et Rhizoma
dà zǎo	大枣	Jujubae, Fructus
dài dài huā	代代花	Citri Aurantii Amarae, Flos
dān shēn	丹参	Salviae Miltiorhizae, Radix
dàn zhú yè	淡竹叶	Lophatheri, Herba
dāng guī	当归	Angelicae Sinensis, Radix
dǎng shēn	党参	Codonopsis, Radix
dì yú	地榆	Sanguisorbae, Radix
dōng guā zī	冬瓜子	Benincasae, Semen
dōng kuí zī	冬葵子	Semen, Malvae
dù héng	杜蘅	Asarum Forbesii (synonym of Heterotropa Forbesii)
dú huó	独活	Angelicae Pubescentis, Radix
ē jiāo	阿胶	Asini Corii, Colla
é zhú	莪术	Curcumae, Rhizoma
ér chá	儿茶	Catechu
fáng fēng	防风	Saposhnikoviae, Radix
fēng mì	蜂蜜	Mel (Honey)
fú líng	茯苓	Poriae Cocos, Sclerotium
fú píng	浮萍	Spirodelae, Herba
gān cǎo	甘草	Glycyrrhizae Uralensis, Radix
gǎo běn	藁本	Ligustici, Rhizoma
gé gēn	葛根	Puerariae, Radix
hǎi dài	海带	Laminariae, Thallus
hǎi zǎo	海藻	Sargassum
hé shǒu wū	何首乌	Polygoni Multiflori, Radix
hēi dòu	黑豆	Sojae Nigrum, Semen
hóng huā	红花	Carthami, Flos
hòu pò	厚朴	Magnoliae Officinalis, Cortex
huá shí	滑石	Talcum
huáng bǎi	黄柏	Phellodendri, Cortex
huáng là	黄蜡	Yellow Wax (Beeswax)

Pīnyīn	Chinese	Pharmaceutical
huáng lián	黄连	Coptidis, Rhizoma
huáng qí	黄芪	Astragali, Radix
huáng qín	黄芩	Scutellariae, Radix
huǒ má rén	火麻仁	Cannabis, Semen
jī guān huā	鸡冠花	Celosiae Cristata, Flos
jiāng cán	僵蚕	Bombyx Batryticatus
jiāng huáng	姜黄	Curcumae Longae, Rhizoma
jiǎo gǔ lán	绞股蓝	Gynostemma Pentaphyllum, Herba
jié gěng	桔梗	Platycodi, Radix
jīn yín huā	金银花	Lonicerae Japonicae, Flos
jīng jiè	荆芥	Schizonepetae, Herba
jīng mǐ	粳米	Oryzae, Semen
jú hóng	桔红	Citri Reticulatae Rubrum, Exocarpium
kǔ shēn	苦参	Sophorae Flavescentis, Radix
kūn bù	昆布	Eckloniae, Thallus
lǎo cōng	老葱	Allii Fistulosi, Bulbus
lǎo hēi cù	老黑醋	Atrum Vetum, Acetum
lián qiáo	连翘	Forsythiae, Fructus
líng xiāo huā	凌霄花	Campsis, Flos
liú huáng	硫磺	Sulphur
lóng dǎn cǎo	龙胆草	Gentianiae, Radix
lòu lú	漏芦	Rhapontici, Radix
lǜ dòu	绿豆	Phaseoli Radiati, Semen
lǜ è méi	绿萼梅	Armeniacae Mume, Flos
lú huì	芦荟	Aloe (dried juice of aloe concentrate)
mǎ chǐ xiàn	马齿苋	Portulacae, Herba
má huáng	麻黄	Ephedrea, Herba
mài mén dōng	麦门冬	Ophiopogonis Japonici, Tuber
máng xiāo	芒硝	Natrii Sulfas
méi guī huā	玫瑰花	Rosae Rugosae, Flos
mì tuó sēng	密陀僧	Lithargyrum
míng fán	明矾	Alumen
mò yào	没药	Myrrha

Pīnyīn	Chinese	Pharmaceutical
mǔ dān pí	牡丹皮	Moutan, Cortex
mù lán pí	木兰皮	Magnolia, Cortex
mǔ lì	牡蛎	Ostrea, Concha
niú huáng	牛黄	Bovis Calculus
niú xī	牛膝	Achyranthis, Radix
pí pá yè	枇杷叶	Eriobotryae Japonicae, Folium
pú gōng yīng	蒲公英	Taraxaci, Herba
qī yè yī zhī huā	七叶一枝花	Paridis, Rhizoma
qiān dān	铅丹	Minium
qiān niú zǐ	牵牛子	Pharbitidis, Semen
qīng dài	青黛	Indigo Naturalis
qīng fěn	轻粉	Calomelas
qīng hāo	青蒿	Artemisiae Annuae, Herba
qīng mù xiāng	青木香	Aristolochiae, Radix
qīng pí	青皮	Citri Reticulatae Viride, Pericarpium
rén shēn	人参	Ginseng, Radix
rǔ xiāng	乳香	Olibanum, Gummi
sān léng	三棱	Sparganii, Rhizoma
sān qī	三七	Notoginseng, Radix
sāng bái pí	桑白皮	Mori, Cortex
shā rén	砂仁	Amomi, Fructus
shān yào	山药	Dioscorea, Rhizome
shān zhā	山楂	Crataegi, Fructus
shān zhū yú	山茱萸	Corni, Fructus
sháo yào	芍药	Paeoniae, Radix
shè xiāng	麝香	Moschus
shēng jiāng	生姜	Zingiberis Recens, Rhizoma
shēng má	升麻	Cimicifugae, Rhizoma
shí chāng pú	石菖蒲	Acori Tatarinowii, Rhizoma
shí gāo	石膏	Gypsum Fibrosum
shú dì huáng	熟地黄	Rehmanniae Preparata, Radix
shuǐ yín	水银	Hydrargyrum
táo rén	桃仁	Persicae, Semen
tiān huā fěn	天花粉	Trichosanthis, Radix

Pīnyīn	Chinese	Pharmaceutical
tiān kuí zǐ	天葵子	Semiaquilegiae, Radix
tiān nán xīng	天南星	Arisaematis, Rhizoma
tǔ fú líng	土茯苓	Smilacis Glabrae, Rhizoma
wǔ bèi zǐ	五倍子	Rhois Chinensis, Galla
wú gōng	蜈蚣	Scolopendra
wú zhū yú	吴茱萸	Evodiae, Fructus
xī huáng shī jiāo	西黄蓍胶	Astragalus, Gummifer
xì xīn	细辛	Asari, Radix
xià kū cǎo	夏枯草	Prunellae Vulgaris, Spica
xìng rén	杏仁	Armeniacae, Semen
xióng huáng	雄黄	Realgar
xuān cǎo huā	萱草花	Hemerocallis Fulva (Day Lily)
xuán shēn	玄参	Scrophulariae Ningpoensis, Radix
xuè jié	血竭	Draconis, Sangusis
yán hú suǒ	延胡索	Cordialis, Rhizoma
yě jú huā	野菊花	Chrysanthemi Indici, Flos
yì mǔ cǎo	益母草	Leonuri, Herba
yì yǐ rén	薏苡仁	Coices, Semen
yīn chén hāo	茵陈蒿	Artemisiae Scopariae, Herba
yú xīng cǎo	鱼腥草	Houttuynia Cordata Thunb., Herba
yù zhú	玉竹	Polygonati Odorati, Rhizoma
zào jiǎo cì	皂角刺	Gleditsiae, Spina
zǎo xiū	蚤休	Paridis, Rhizoma
zé lán	泽兰	Lycopi, Herba
zé xiè	泽泻	Alismatis, Rhizoma
zhāng nǎo	樟脑	Camphora
zhè bèi mǔ	浙贝母	Fritillariae Thunbergii, Bulbus
zhēn zhū mǔ	珍珠母	Margaritaferae, Concha
zhì bàn xià	制半夏	Pinelliae Preparatum, Rhizoma
zhì gān cǎo	炙甘草	Glycyrrhizae Preparata, Radix
zhǐ ké	枳壳	Citri Aurantii, Fructus
zhī má yóu	芝麻油	Sesame Oil
zhī mǔ	知母	Anemarrhenae, Rhizoma
zhī zǐ	栀子	Gardeniae, Fructus

Pīnyīn	Chinese	Pharmaceutical
zǐ cǎo	紫草	Arnebiae Seu Lithospermi, Radix
zǐ huā dì dīng	紫花地丁	Violae, Herba

Appendix IV: Historical and Source Text Bibliography

Pīnyīn title	Chinese title	English title	Author (English)	Author (Chinese)	Published
Dòng Tiān Ào Zhǐ	洞天奥旨	Secrets of External Medicine	Chén Shì-Duó	陈世铎	17th–18th century
Gǔ Jīn Yī Tǒng Dà Quán	古今医统大全	The Complete Compendium of Ancient and Modern Medical Works	Xú Chūn-Fǔ	徐春甫	1556
Huáng Dì Nèi Jīng	黄帝内经	The Inner Canon of the Yellow Emperor	Unknown	未知	Between the late Warring States period and the Hàn Dynasty
Mài Jué Xin Biān	脉诀新编	New Version of Pulse Diagnosis	Liú Běn-Chāng	刘本昌	1939
Nèi Kē Zhāi Yào	内科摘要	Summary of Internal Medicine	Xuē Jǐ	薛己	1529
Pǔ Jì Fāng	普济方	Prescriptions for Universal Relief	Zhū Sù *et al.*	朱橚等	1406
Pǔ Jì Fāng Xīn Biān Tóu Miàn Bù Jí Bìng	普济方新编头面部疾病	New Version of Pu Jifang's Head and Face Diseases	Guō Zhì-Huá, Xiào Guó-Shì	郭志华,肖国士	2012
Qiān Jīn Yì Fāng	千金翼方	Supplement to Important Formulas Worth a Thousand Gold Pieces	Sūn Sī-Miǎo	孙思邈	682
Shāng Hán Zá Bìng Lùn	伤寒杂病论	Treatise on Cold Damage Diseases and Miscellaneous Diseases	Zhāng Zhòng-Jīng	张仲景	c. 219 AD

Pīnyīn title	Chinese title	English title	Author (English)	Author (Chinese)	Published
Shén Nóng Běn Cǎo Jīng Jí Zhù	神农本草经集注	Collected Commentaries on Shén Nóng's Materia Medica	Táo Hóng-Jǐng	陶弘景	6th century
Shèng Jì Zōng Lù	圣济总录	Comprehensive Recording of Sacred Relief	Northern Sòng Government (Physicians of the Sòng Imperial Court)	北宋政府	1111–1118
Shòu Shì Bǎo Yuán	寿世保元	Prolonging Life and Preserving the Origin	Gōng Tíng-Xián	龚廷贤	1615
Sù Wèn Bìng Jī Qì Yí Bǎo Mìng Jí	素问病机气宜保命集	Collection of Writings on the Mechanism of Disease, Suitability of Qì, and the Safeguarding of Life as Discussed in the "Basic Questions"	Liú Wán-Sù	刘完素	1186
Tài Píng Huì Mín Hé Jì Jú Fāng	太平惠民和剂局方	Formulary of the Pharmacy Service for Benefiting the People in the Taiping Era	Imperial Medical Bureau	太医局	1107–1110
Tài Píng Shèng Huì Fāng	太平圣惠方	Taiping Holy Prescriptions for Universal Relief	Wáng Huái-Yǐn	王怀隐	Completed 992 AD
Wài Kē Dà Chéng	外科大成	Great Compendium of External Medicine	Qí Kūn	祁坤	1665
Wài Kē Jīng Yào	外科精要	Essence of Diagnosis and Treatment of External Diseases	Chén Zì-Míng	陈自明	1263
Wài Kē Jīng Yì	外科精义	Treatment of Surgical Diseases	Qí Dé-Zhī	齐德之	1335
Wài Kē Lǐ Lì	外科理例	Exemplars for Applying the Principles of External Medicine	Wāng Jī	汪机	1531
Wài Kē Qǐ Xuán	外科启玄	Profound Insights on External Diseases	Shēn Dǒu-Yuán	申斗垣	1604

Pīnyīn title	Chinese title	English title	Author (English)	Author (Chinese)	Published
Wài Kē Zhēn Quán	外科真诠	Personal Experience in *Wài Kē*	Zōu Yuè	邹岳	1838
Wài Kē Zhèng Zhì Quán Shēng Jí	外科证治全生集	Complete Compendium of Patterns and Treatments in External Medicine	Wáng Wéi-Dé	王维德	1740
Wài Kē Zhèng Zhì Quán Shū	外科证治全书	Complete Book of Patterns and Treatments in External Medicine	Xǔ Kè-Chāng	许克昌	1831
Wài Kē Zhèng Zōng	外科正宗	True Lineage of External Medicine	Chén Shí-Gōng	陈实功	1617
Wài Tài Mì Yào	外台秘要	Arcane Essentials from the Imperial Library	Wáng Tāo	王焘	752
Wàn Bìng Huí Chūn	万病回春	The Restoration of Health from the Myriad Diseases	Gǒng Tíng-Xián	龚廷贤	1587
Wāng Shíshān Yī Shū Bā Zhǒng	汪石山医书八种	Wāng Shíshān's Eight Medical Books	Wāng Jī	汪机	1522–1633
Yāng Shēng Fāng	养生方	Formulas for Nourishing Life	Unknown	未知	202 BC–8 AD
Yī Jīng Yuán Zhǐ	医经原旨	The Original Meaning of Medical Classics	Xuē Xuě	薛雪	1754
Yī Lěi Yuán Róng	医垒元戎	Supreme Commanders of the Medical Ramparts	Wáng Hào-Gǔ	王好古	1291
Yī Lín Gǎi Cuò	医林改错	Corrections of Errors Among Physicians	Wáng Qīng-Rèn	王清任	1830
Yī Xué Gāng Mù	医学纲目	The Grand Compendium of Medicine	Lóu Yīng	楼英	c. 1320–1389
Yī Zōng Jīn Jiàn	医宗金鉴	The Golden Mirror of Ancestral Medicine	Wú Qiān *et al.*	吴谦等	c. 1736–1743

Pīnyīn title	Chinese title	English title	Author (English)	Author (Chinese)	Published
Zhào Bǐng-Nán Lín Chuáng Jīng Yàn Jí	赵炳南临床经验集	Zhào Bǐng-Nán's Clinical Experience Set	Zhào Bǐng-Nán	赵炳南	1975
Zhēn Jiǔ Féng Yuán	针灸逢原	Encountering the Sources of Acupuncture and Moxibustion	Lǐ Xué-Chuān	李学川	1817
Zhōng Guó Zhōng Yī Mì Fāng Dà Quán	中国中医秘方大全	The Complete Compendium of Secret Chinese TCM Formulas	Hú Xī-Míng	胡熙明	1989
Zhōng Yī Wài Kē Xué	中医外科学	Traditional Chinese Medicine Surgery	Zhū Rén-Kāng	朱仁康	1987
Zhǒu Hòu Bèi Jí Fāng	肘后备急方	Emergency Formulas to Keep Up One's Sleeve	Gě Hóng	葛洪	3rd century
Zhū Bìng Yuán Hóu Lùn	诸病源侯论	General Treatise on the Etiology and Symptomology of Diseases	Cháo Yuán-Fāng	巢元方	610
Zhū Rén Kāng Lín Chuáng Jīng Yàn Jí	朱仁康临床经验集	A Collection of Zhu Rén-Kāng's Clinical Experiences	Zhū Rén-Kāng	朱仁康	1979
[Zhù Shì] Huáng Dì Nèi Jīng Sù Wèn	(注释)黄帝内经素问	Annotations on The Yellow Emperor's Inner Classic	Wáng Bīng	王冰	762 AD

Subject Index

Herb Index

Formula Index